Profiles and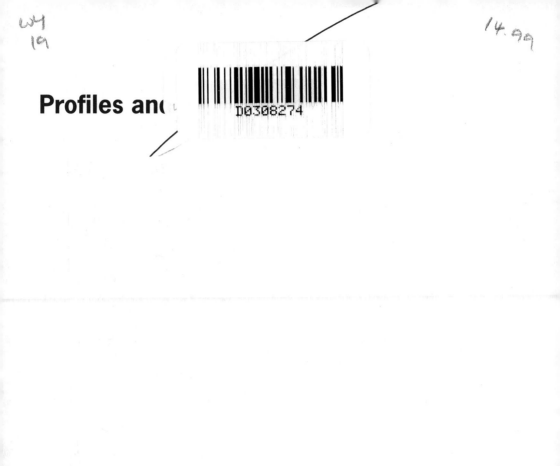

D0308274

Profiles and Portfolios

A Guide for Health and Social Care

Second Edition

Cathy Hull, Liz Redfern and Ann Shuttleworth

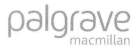

First editon 1996
Second edition 2005
Published by
PALGRAVE MACMILLAN
Houndmills, Basingstoke, Hampshire RG21 6XS and
175 Fifth Avenue, New York, N.Y. 10010
Companies and representatives throughout the world

PALGRAVE MACMILLAN is the global academic imprint of the Palgrave Macmillan division of St. Martin's Press, LLC and of Palgrave Macmillan Ltd. Macmillan® is a registered trademark in the United States, United Kingdom and other countries. Palgrave is a registered trademark in the European Union and other countries.

ISBN 1–4039–1509–1

This book is printed on paper suitable for recycling and made from fully managed and sustained forest sources.

A catalogue record for this book is available from the British Library.

10 9 8 7 6 5 4 3 2 1
14 13 12 11 10 09 08 07 06 05

Printed in Great Britain by
Creative Print & Design (Wales), Ebbw Vale

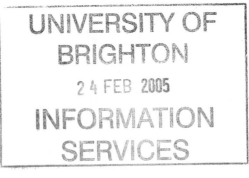

This book is dedicated to Vernon, Tiny, Mike, Harold and Jean
for being there

The Companion Website

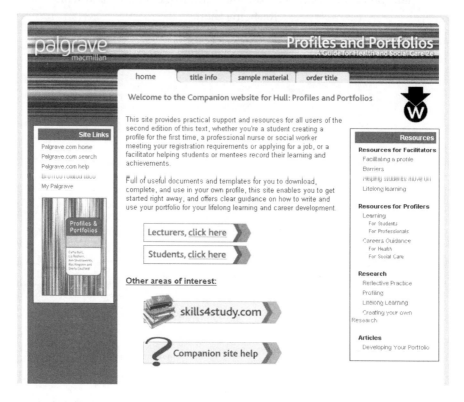

A profile or portfolio is a record of learning and achievement, an essential tool for professional development, and a statutory requirement for all health and social care professionals. Get started on yours right now by visiting www.palgrave.com/hull. Full of useful advice, documents, templates, practical support and resources, the companion website offers clear guidance on how to write and use your portfolio for your lifelong learning and career development.

Complete with careers guidance, learning resources and research tips, the *Profiles and Portfolios* companion website is a valuable resource to be used alongside the text, whether you're a lecturer, student, professional or researcher.

Contents

List of Table and Figures   x
Acknowledgements   xi
Introduction   xiii

1   Profiles and Portfolios: The Health Care Context   **1**
Influences on the development of profiles   2
Statutory bodies   2
Reflective practice   5
Adult and higher education   6
Market forces   7
Uses within health care   10
PREP requirements   10
Job applications   10
Identifying personal goals   11
Focus for organising your own learning   11
Supporting learning from practice and clinical supervision   12
Tool for reflective practice   12
Achieving credit as part of a prior learning claim   12
Assessment for an educational programme   13
Lifelong learning   13
References   15

2   Profiles and Portfolios: The Social Care Context   **16**
Evidence-based practice, lifelong learning and portfolio
    development   18
Standards for social care   19
Occupational standards for social care   19
Continuing professional development   21
References   22

3   Getting to Grips with the Terminology   **23**
Lifelong learning   23
Lifelong learning and work   24
Continuing professional development   26
Profiles and portfolios   28
Experiential learning   30
Reflection   32

Learning outcomes   33
Multidisciplinary teams: the challenge for CPD   34
Progress files and personal development planning   34
Credit frameworks   35
Key skills   35
Glossary of terms   36
References   36

4 Some Common Themes and Questions Shared   **37**
Why do I need to compile a profile?   38
Should I buy a ready-made profile?   39
How do I decide which profile to buy?   39
What can I put into it?   43
How long will it take to complete?   44
Who owns my profile?   44
How do I know that the learning I am demonstrating is
at the appropriate level?   44
How much information should I include?   45
What should I do if I haven't written for a long time?   45
Where can I go for help?   46
References   47

5 Getting Started: Creating Your Personal Profile   **48**
Taking stock   49
Developing a structure   58
Reflecting on past learning   60
Identifying significant learning   61
Proving what you know and can do   66
Constructing your profile   70
References   75

6 Profiles and Reflective Practice   **76**
Role of reflection in professional practice   77
Reflection and learning   78
Defining reflection and reflective practice   80
Reflection and profiles   81
Writing and reflecting   82
Confidentiality   83
Reflection – how do you do it?   85
Ideas for further work on reflection   91
References   92

7   **Making Your Learning Count**   **94**
     Towards a definition of accreditation   95
     Accreditation of continuing professional development   96
     National Occupational Standards   96
     National Vocational Qualifications   97
     Key skills   99
     Awarding bodies   99
     National Qualifications Framework   100
     Accreditation and your portfolio   101
     Other awarding bodies   107

8   **Helping Others to Develop a Profile: The Skills of**
     Facilitation   **108**
     Learning from experience   108
     Assisting others with their profile   112
     Blocks to learning   113
     Facilitation skills   115
     Planning the profile   118
     Establishing ground rules   122
     Progress chasing   123
     Evaluation   123
     References   124

9   **Further Resources: Further Activities to Help You Develop**
     Your Profile   **125**
     Activity 1: Conducting a personal SWOT analysis   125
     Activity 2: Mind mapping   130
     Activity 3. Goal and action planning   132
     Activity 4: Understanding your learning style   133
     PEST analysis   137
     Goal and action plan form   140
     References   141

Annotated Bibliography   142
Index   151

List of Tables and Figures

Tables

7.1   National Vocational Qualification Framework   98
7.2   National Credit Framework   99
7.3   Equivalences between WN Credit Framework levels
      and other qualifications   100
7.4   National Qualifications Framework   101

Figures

3.1   Types of personal portfolio   29
5.1   Documenting experience   60
5.2   The development process   61
5.3   Example showing how development through the profile
      process can be related to the learning cycle   65
6.1   Kolb's learning cycle   78
6.2   Gibbs' reflective cycle   79
6.3   Sheckley and Keeton's learning cycle   79
8.1   Kolb's learning cycle (adapted)   109

Acknowledgements

This book would not have been possible without the opportunity we have had to share, discuss and develop our ideas with people who know about the issues, or are interested in learning. If we had included everyone we would have filled the whole book. We would therefore like to thank the following for their generosity of spirit, knowledge, encouragement and time: Joanna Price, Jennifer Wyatt, Chris James, Helen Hume, Krysia Hudek.

Introduction

In the last few years, the terms 'profile' and 'portfolio' have become familiar to nurses, midwives and health visitors. They are expected to keep a profile to document their professional development in order to remain on the professional register that gives them permission to practise. The terms are also becoming familiar to social workers and health and social care assistants, who are increasingly required to keep profiles while on educational courses. They are not legally required to keep a profile at the moment, but this may change in the future.

The idea for developing the first edition of this book came from our experience of speaking at nursing conferences and running workshops, and our direct involvement in helping nurses, midwives and health visitors to understand and put together profiles.

Our experience led us to realise that although people who are familiar with the terms quickly grasp the idea that profiling can help them in their professional development, they then do not know how to start. They are unsure of the practical issues, such as how to develop a profile and how they can relate it to their practice. This uncertainty caused many nurses, midwives and health visitors sleepless nights. The requirement to maintain a profile in order to remain on the professional register meant they worried that they may be struck off if they did not do it properly, and would therefore lose their careers and livelihoods.

Since the first edition of the book was published, profiling has become relevant to more people working in health and social care. Although they do not currently have a professional register, health care assistants and social care assistants are increasingly required to gain National Vocational Qualifications, and are expected to keep a profile as part of their coursework. Social workers do have a professional register and, like nurses, midwives and health visitors, will soon be required to undertake continuing professional development in order to remain on the register. The principles and practicalities of keeping a profile are generally the same for all professions. In revising and updating this book, we have therefore expanded its scope to make it relevant to health and social care assistants and social workers and thus to enable them to develop their own profiles.

The common questions people ask when seeking advice about profiles are:

- Do I need to buy one?
- If I do, which one is likely to meet my needs?

- Can I develop one on my own, or do I need help?
- How can I express my life and work experience in a containable and meaningful way?
- Where do I start?

This book aims to help people to answer these questions for themselves by giving practical guidance on the whole profiling process, from start to finish – although accepting that once you have developed a profile, maintaining it is a neverending process. The book is based on what we think people need to know to make a success of profiling and, more importantly, includes information on the issues they ask for help with.

The book will give you guidance in compiling your own profile, and is intended to support you in the process rather than to provide a model profile. Different formats will suit different people, so we aim to help you to decide what will work for you and enable you to meet your own needs and those of your regulatory body, educational institution or employer. Although we suggest activities and include an annotated bibliography of resource material that will help you with the process, this is not a book you are expected to work through from start to finish, using the activities to create your profile. It is intended to support the process rather than to dictate to you how to do it.

Readers will bring their own styles and learning needs to the book, so you should use it in the way that works best for you. We have written it knowing that most people will dip in and out of it when they have particular learning needs. Each chapter therefore has a brief section explaining what it contains, so you can decide whether it is relevant for you at the time. However, the chapters do follow a logical sequence, so you can read the book from cover to cover and gain a picture of the development and the process of profiling if you wish.

You may be aware that the terms 'profile' and 'portfolio' are used interchangeably in health and social care. This issue is addressed in several chapters, so we will not repeat the arguments here. However, we have decided to use the term profile unless we are referring to a specific product known as a portfolio.

The book has combined the experiences of three people from different backgrounds. Cathy Hull has a background in adult education, experiential processes and facilitating others in the profiling process from outside health and social care. Liz Redfern brings her experience of profiles and reflective practice from a professional context of nursing and midwifery practice and education. Ann Shuttleworth has a background in professional publishing in health and social care. We believe that our different backgrounds have enabled us to make the book a practical and informative resource that will help a range of health and social care professionals to get to grips with profiling. We hope it will also show you that there is no mystery in the process, and that it should not be the cause of worry and anxiety. Once you understand what you need to achieve and have got under way, profiling should not be difficult or too time-consuming. It can become an integral part of your working life, and can make many aspects of it easier for you by helping you to learn from your experience, identify your learning needs and demonstrate to others what you have learned. In the long run, it may actually save you time, and should help you to develop your career and earning potential.

So what does the book contain? The following chapter-by-chapter break-down gives an overview.

Chapter 1   Profiles and Portfolios: The Health Care Context
This chapter charts the history of profiling in health care, and identifies the factors, such as statutory bodies, reflective practice, market forces and educational institutions, that have influenced the introduction of profiling in health care. It aims to demonstrate why profiling is relevant to health care professionals, and how they can use it to develop their career.

Chapter 2   Profiles and Portfolios: The Social Care Context
This chapter charts the development of profiling in social care. Like Chapter 1 it looks at the different factors influencing the introduction of profiling and explains its relevance to social care professionals.

Chapter 3   Getting to Grips with the Terminology
This chapter attempts to unravel the confusion in terminology, so that everyone can understand it and use it appropriately.

Chapter 4   Some Common Themes and Questions Shared
Here we explore the 10 most common questions asked about profiles.

Chapter 5   Getting Started: Creating Your Personal Profile
In this chapter you will find practical advice and activities on how to develop a framework for a profile to meet your individual needs.

Chapter 6   Profiles and Reflective Practice
This chapter attempts to demystify the concept of reflective practice and offers some practical strategies for beginners.

Chapter 7   Making Your Learning Count
This chapter will be helpful if you are developing a profile to seek accreditation within an educational programme or system.

Chapter 8   Helping Others to Develop a Profile: The Skills of Facilitation
In this chapter, we look at some of the specific skills you will need to help someone else to complete a profile. We look at how adults learn and explore the five key skills of facilitation. It is written with practitioners in mind, but might also be useful for teachers.

Further Resources: Further Activities to Help You Develop Your Profile
We realised it would be helpful for readers to have access to resources that will help them with the profiling process. This resource material comes from several disciplines.

Profiles and Portfolios: The Health Care Context

This chapter charts the history and identifies the factors that have influenced the introduction of profiles into the world of health care, focusing on nurses, midwives and health visitors, and health care assistants. It discusses some of the uses that have been identified for profiles in health care, and the benefits health care professionals can gain from developing and using a profile. Finally it looks briefly at developments within health care that add to the importance of using profiles.

All nurses, midwives and health visitors on the professional register have been required for some time to use a profile or portfolio to maintain their registration. The requirement was introduced in the 1990s by the profession's governing body of the time, the United Kingdom Central Council for Nursing, Midwifery and Health Visiting (UKCC) as part of its Post-Registration Education and Practice (PREP) initiative. This requires all practitioners to undertake continuing professional development (CPD). Their Personal Professional Portfolios are used to demonstrate that individual practitioners have fulfilled their PREP requirements in order to remain on the register.

Although health care assistants do not have a statutory requirement to use a profile, those who are undertaking NVQ courses need to do so to demonstrate their learning. This chapter sets the scene by identifying the factors that have influenced the increasing use of profiles in health care. While practitioners have to maintain profiles in order to meet their professional or educational requirements, there are other reasons for doing so. We hope this book will help you to understand why profiles can help you in your personal and professional development. Even if you do not currently need to use a profile for professional or educational reasons, we hope it will show you why it is a good idea and how it may help you in the future.

Influences on the development of profiles

Articles about the use of portfolios began to appear in the nursing and mid-wifery press in the early 1990s. However, like most major changes in professional behaviour, it is difficult to pinpoint exactly who started the ball rolling or when. The process was gradual, and was influenced by a number of factors such as:

- The requirements of statutory bodies
- The recognition that reflective practice can help professionals to develop their practice
- Market forces
- The requirements of educational institutions.

Statutory bodies

Statutory bodies have been influential in introducing the concept of profiles, and continue to support their use. This is interesting, because these bodies often lag behind the profession in educational and professional development, because of their necessarily slow decision-making processes. In the case of nursing, midwifery and health visiting, however, the professional body took a lead by making it a statutory requirement for professionals to use a profile.

The UKCC introduced the requirement for all registrants to use a portfolio in 1995. This was part of the introduction of PREP, which made it a statutory requirement for practitioners to undertake CPD within each three-year registration period. Each time they apply to renew their registration, practitioners must be able to show that they have fulfilled their responsibilities, which are set out in two PREP standards:

The PREP (practice) standard   This requires practitioners to undertake at least 100 days (or 750 hours) of professional practice in the previous five years;

The PREP (continuing professional development) standard   This requires practitioners to have undertaken and recorded at least five days (or 35 hours) of CPD in the previous three-year registration period.

Profiles – or Personal Professional Portfolios – were introduced as the method by which nurses and midwives could demonstrate that they had met the CPD standard. They had a few years to get used to the idea and to develop their portfolios, but in 2000 practitioners were required to declare on their Notification of Practice form that they had met this requirement when they applied to renew their registration. The following year the UKCC began to audit compliance with the CPD standard. In 2002 the UKCC was replaced by the Nursing and Midwifery Council (NMC). The council also took over the functions of the four National Boards and continues to audit the CPD standard. Each month, up to 10 per cent of those applying to renew their registration are issued with PREP (CPD) summary forms. These are sent out between 14 and 90 days before their renewal date, and ask registrants to give a brief description of the CPD they have undertaken and its relevance to their work. The forms must be returned to the NMC before registration can be renewed. Midwives had been required to undertake CPD for some time before the introduction of PREP under Rule 37 of the Midwives Rules. In 2001, however, this was superseded by the PREP standards, bringing midwifery in line with nursing and health visiting. In order to help practitioners to make sense of their PREP requirements, the NMC has issued *The PREP Handbook* (NMC, 2002), which sets out in detail what it expects.

The handbook makes it clear that the CPD standard can be fulfilled in many ways. The important thing is that practitioners record all learning activities in their Personal Professional Portfolio, so that when they come to renew their registration they have a clear record of all CPD activities they have undertaken and how their practice benefited as a result.

The handbook also gives a number of case studies showing different ways of recording CPD and the different types of activities that are considered relevant. It clearly shows that the process of demonstrating fulfilment of the CPD standard is not complicated. However, without a Personal Professional Portfolio with clear records of CPD activities to refer back to, the task would be far more difficult!

The PREP Handbook makes the following points about CPD that are useful to remember:

- It does not have to cost any money.
- There is no such thing as approved PREP (CPD) activity.
- You don't need to collect points or certificates of attendance.
- There is no approved format for the Personal Professional Portfolio.
- It must be relevant to the work you are doing and/or plan to do in the near future.
- It must help you to provide the highest possible standards of care for your patients.

Because there is no approved format for the Personal Professional Portfolio, it is up to individual practitioners to develop their own in a form that suits them. In order for it to be as useful as possible, however, it should be a reflective document, showing how reflection has helped the practitioner to make sense of learning – both through CPD and day-to-day practice.

We will discuss reflective practice on page 5 and in greater detail in Chapter 6. Although they no longer exist, two of the National Boards did play an important role in influencing and increasing professional awareness and understanding of the use of profiles and portfolios. Even before the introduction of PREP, the Welsh National Board produced a Professional Profile Folder, which it made available in 1991. This used a similar format to personal organisers, which were becoming widely used at the time. Many practitioners have found this a useful way of keeping a profile or portfolio, as it enables them to keep material in clearly defined sections for ease of reference.

Soon after, the English National Board produced a framework for continuing professional education (ENB, 1991), which has helped many practitioners to clarify what constitutes CPD. The framework was designed around 10 key characteristics of professional practice, which are said to represent the benchmarks of expert professional practice and remain relevant today – not only to nurses, midwives and health visitors, but to all health care professionals. These key characteristics relate to:

- Professional accountability and responsibility
- Clinical expertise with a specific client group
- Use of research to plan, implement and evaluate strategies to improve care
- Teamworking and building, and multidisciplinary team leadership
- Flexible and innovative approaches to care
- Use of health promotion strategies
- Facilitating and assessing development in others
- Handling information and making informed clinical decisions
- Setting standards and evaluating quality of care
- Initiating, managing and evaluating clinical change.

Although the framework ceased to operate when the NMC replaced the ENB, these key characteristics can be helpful in planning your CPD – if your learning activities fulfil one or more of the characteristics it is relevant to your PREP requirements.

Terminology

Some readers may be wondering about our apparently inconsistent use of terminology to describe profiles and portfolios in this chapter. We have used different terms such as 'Personal Professional Portfolio' and 'Professional Profile Folder' as they are or were applied by the different statutory bodies. So, the NMC refers to a Personal Professional Portfolio, but in our experience, the terms 'profile' and 'portfolio' are used interchangeably, and often inaccurately.

Chapter 3 discusses the terminology associated with profiles and portfolios in some detail. At this point terminology is not important except to note that within health care there seems to be some confusion and inconsistency. From now on we will use the term profile unless we are talking about a specific product that calls itself a portfolio.

Reflective practice

While the use of profiles was growing in nursing and midwifery, a parallel development was the growing acknowledgement of reflective practice as a tool in professional development. We will discuss reflective practice in more detail in Chapter 6, but here we will discuss it in the context of its influence on profiles.

Any readers who have recently completed a nursing or midwifery course at either pre-registration or post-registration level are likely to have been asked to complete a reflective journal or diary. Some NVQ students may also be asked to do this. Most commercially available profiles encourage their owners to reflect, and to use the profile to store the outcomes of the reflective process. Some also give advice on how to develop skills in reflection.

By encouraging reflective practice, profiles generate further interest in reflective practice. Equally, since reflective practitioners need to write about their reflections, reflective practice encourages the use of profiles, which are the ideal place to do this. However, even if you have a commercially developed profile that gives advice on reflection, it is unlikely to be comprehensive, and you are likely to need to supplement it with further reading on the subject of reflection and reflective practice. Chapter 6 is a good place to start.

Professionals often express concern about how confidential and secure a record of reflective practice can be within a profile. Once you have committed the outcomes of your reflections to paper or computer disc, who does it belong to? Who has the right to see it? There have been some occasions where the contents of personal diaries or reflective journals have been subpoenaed as evidence within cases of professional conduct or litigation.

Confidentiality is a difficult issue when it comes to reflection. In most situations, you can keep sections of your reflective writings just for yourself, and should not be expected to show it to anyone else. You may need to generate sections that demonstrate how your reflections have helped your professional development and that you are happy to show to others such as tutors and managers, but it is quite normal to have a 'private' section.

However, in cases where you are called upon to give evidence, a court or disciplinary committee may require these private sections. Of course, you need to remember that in such a situation you would in any case be expected to tell 'the truth, the whole truth and nothing but the truth' as a law-abiding citizen, so it should not be a problem to show your reflective journal. You may even find the journal helpful in jogging your memory, since hearings often happen months after the incident in question.

This requirement to tell the truth means that even if you do not write about an incident in your reflective journal, you may be asked to give evidence about it. Just because you did not write about an incident does not mean it did not happen, so you could still be asked to give verbal evidence about it.

Putting aside the spectre of giving evidence for a moment, under normal circumstances you have a choice about what you record in your reflective diary and profile. You also have a choice about what parts you share, when and with whom. The issue of confidentiality is discussed in more detail in Chapter 6.

We believe the outcomes of reflective practice and the learning that occurs as a result is professional knowledge in the making. In the past nurses, midwives and other professionals depended on information in textbooks and articles to help them to know what to do and when. However, this knowledge can also be developed through the insight gained during reflective practice, which has the benefit of being grounded in clinical practice, and therefore relevant to your work. Journals and books are increasingly using reflective material, for example in the form of case examples in which the author or another practitioner discusses a case and reflects on how it might influence their practice in future.

Adult and higher education

The development and use of profiles within health care has been heavily influenced by educationalists in adult and higher education. The professional preparation these people received in order to become teachers, tutors or lecturers has made them aware of the ways in which profiles are used in other contexts, both within health care and other spheres. These applications include:

- as a profile approach to assessment
- as part of a claim for prior learning within a credit accumulation and transfer scheme
- the use of learning contracts within profiles
- the student-centred approach that profiles encourage.

Many educationalists working in health care also find the use of profiles attractive because is enables students to take an open learning approach, where they identify their own learning needs. This enables educationalists to become facilitators, encouraging students' professional development and helping them to define and meet their learning needs, rather than simply teaching all students the same material, regardless of their learning needs and prior knowledge and experience.

Market forces

When the use of Personal Professional Portfolios became a statutory requirement for nurses, midwives and health visitors on the register, a number of publishing houses produced profiles. The quality and approach of these commercially produced profiles varied – particularly since the UKCC at the time did not give rigid instructions as to what format they should take.

A number are still available, both for nurses and midwives and for health care assistants. While practitioners are free to develop their profiles as they see fit, many find it helpful to have a ready-made structure to follow or to adapt to suit themselves. Many also find it helpful to have advice and guidance contained within the profile.

If you have not already bought a commercially available profile for your own use, this book should help you to understand more about why and how you might use one. It should therefore help you to decide whether you want to buy a profile or develop your own, and to evaluate the commercially available ones to see which is best for you. Chapter 4 gives more information on this subject.

Some commercially available profiles are little more than ring binders with dividers and a place to record personal and professional details. Others help you to develop self-awareness and reflective skills. For example, Unison (2001), the public sector union, has developed *The HCA*

Profile: A Personal Development Pack, which is designed to help health care assistants to identify and clarify their skills, knowledge, values and beliefs, aiming to help with both personal and professional development. Yet more are linked to specific CPD programmes, and are driven as much by educational and commercial considerations. *The Profile Pack*, developed by Emap Healthcare Open Learning (1994), links with EHOL's open learning programmes, which can be undertaken in partnership with a number of universities. Some educational institutions have also developed profiles, which are usually sold to students. Some practitioners are understandably unsure whether they can develop their own profile, or whether to buy a ready-made product. The answer is that it depends what suits the individual. Provided a profile meets the requirements of the relevant professional body or educational institution, it does not matter whether it is home-made or off-the-shelf.

One criticism of ready-made profiles is that they look too smart. Some people have said they are apprehensive about writing in them for fear of making them look untidy. Many users do prefer to keep such profiles for special occasions, such as to show at a job interview or for a presentation of their work. It is true that one file or folder is unlikely to be enough to hold all the information and observations you will acquire over your professional life. It may therefore be a good idea to have a 'special' profile folder to keep information you are likely to want to 'show off' whether or not this is a commercially available profile.

You may also find it useful to keep a pocket-size notebook to jot down observations and reflections quickly during your working day or when you get home. This will need to be reviewed from time to time, which is a useful time to decide what you want to transfer into a more permanent file.

The NMC website contains some useful information about the requirements of profiles for nurses and midwives, some of which will also be helpful to health care assistants. The NMC says that there are three broad steps involved in developing a profile:

Reviewing experience to date

Think about what you have done so far, particularly in the past three years. Identify the areas of practice you enjoy most and do well, and those you may need to improve. Think about what you have done to improve your practice and how you intend to continue to do so. Consider relevant areas outside your practice, such as team leadership.

Self-appraisal

Based on the above review, step back and appraise your performance and standards of knowledge and practice. It may help to focus on one event and to analyse critically what happened to and around you at the time. This event could be something that went well or badly. Describe what happened, identify what you learned and consider areas for professional development thrown up by the event. You may find it helpful to discuss the event with a manager or supervisor to focus your thoughts.

Setting goals and action plans

Once you have identified your learning needs you can start setting goals and developing action plans to help you to meet these needs, and evaluating the outcomes. Although self-appraisal should be a continuous process, it is particularly important to appraise your performance if you change your job, undertake an assignment or course, or are involved in a significant event.

The NMC leaves it to individuals to decide how they organise all this information. It says the main considerations to bear in mind are that it should be flexible, accessible and confidential – no patients, clients or carers should be identified in your profile. It also recommends that practitioners consider dividing the profile into two sections, one containing confidential information, the other containing material the NMC may require for audit purposes.

While registered nurses and midwives are free to develop their profiles as they see fit in order to fulfil their PREP (CPD) standard, those on particular courses may be asked to follow guidelines to meet the requirements of their course. This is also true for health care assistants undertaking NVQ training. For example, Guernsey's Institute of Health Studies provides NVQ training in Care at levels 2 and 3. Its website (www.cwgsy.net/community/mindinfo/nvq.htm) states that students' portfolios should contain the following:

- Contents page – with item numbers
- Witness status list
- National standards (copies of units, elements – performance criteria, etc.)
- Assessment plan
- Action plans (at least 2)
- Feedback reports (at least 2)
- Direct observations (at least 2)
- Witness testimonies (at least 2)
- Pre-set written questions and answers
- Other evidence
- All items of evidence must include the candidate's name, candidate number and date.

Uses within health care

You will have your own reasons for picking up this book – perhaps you want to know more about profiles in general, or you may have been prompted for a more specific purpose. While profiles are most widely used in CPD, enabling nurses and midwives to fulfil their PREP requirements, they are increasingly used in education and training. So, perhaps you are on a pre-registration nursing or midwifery course and want to get into the habit of using a portfolio, are undertaking NVQ training in care and want advice about how to develop your profile.

Whatever your reasons for picking up the book, it is likely that you will start using a profile for a particular reason, then broaden your use as you find that you can do more with it. For example, in 1995 the ENB demonstrated that profiles have many uses suggesting that they could be used as:

- a record of professional experience, therefore contributing to PREP requirements
- part of the process of applying for jobs
- part of individual performance review (IPR), helping to identify personal goals and how these are to be achieved
- a focus for organising individual learning
- a way to support learning from practice and clinical supervision
- a tool for reflective practice
- a means of achieving accreditation as part of a prior learning claim
- a way of demonstrating learning for assessment towards educational programmes.

PREP requirements

We have already discussed the NMC's PREP requirements for nurses and midwives to maintain a Personal Professional Profile. You can obtain more details of its requirements and how to fulfil them in *The PREP Handbook*. This is available free from the NMC at 23 Portland Place, London W1N 4QT, or you can download it from the NMC website (www.nmc-uk.org/cms/content/publication – in the section on Registration).

Job applications

It is now common, particularly if you are applying for a more senior post, to be asked to supply a curriculum vitae (CV) to accompany or replace the traditional job application forms. If you keep records of all your educational qualifications and work experience in your profile you will certainly find it easier to construct your CV, and to keep it up to date. Expecting to remember details about courses months or years later, or to find elusive bits of paper can be a frustrating experience. By keeping everything together in your profile you can avoid this. You may find that it is worth adapting your CV to suit a particular job application, emphasising your experience and skills that are most relevant.

Some people now take their whole profile to job interviews. However, it is worth checking beforehand whether the employer requires this level of information. Most expect candidates to pick out experiences from their past career that have a particular bearing on the current job application. It may therefore be better simply to read through your profile before the interview to refresh your memory.

Identifying personal goals

Most staff in health care now experience some form of IPR. Each employer will have its own system for assessing and reviewing an employee's performance, and the frequency of reviews also varies. However, most IPR systems include an opportunity for you to look back on the previous review period and identify achievements and disappointments. They also have a section where you are asked to look forward to the forthcoming period and identify what personal development needs you may have to enable you to fulfil your role or to progress towards a more senior role. This process of looking back and thinking forward can be much easier if you have maintained a profile, as it is likely to contain details of formal or informal learning opportunities you have had during the review period. Your reflections on critical incidents will identify areas where you feel particularly confident and those where you may need further training or support. All this information can be extremely useful when completing a self-assessment exercise as part of the IPR paperwork.

Focus for organising your own learning

When you are enrolled on a particular course or programme of study or training, it is easier to organise your learning agenda around the demands of the course. However, this is not always the case when you are simply doing your job – you are working hard and have no particular focus for your learning or reason for writing about it. Keeping a profile can give you a focus for learning in a number of ways.

- It can store relevant articles and references.
- You can write regular notes about what you have learnt and what you need to find out more about.
- You can record the outcomes of any self-assessment and what you need to do to act on these.

Using a profile in this way means you have to discipline yourself to review its contents on a regular basis. This helps you to make sense of the contents – to see where you have been, say, over the past three months. Looking back on a range of experiences in this way can be a useful springboard to knowing what needs to happen next on your learning pathway. It can also be a great confidence booster, as it helps you to realise how much you have achieved and how much you are capable of.

Supporting learning from practice and clinical supervision

The points to be made here are very similar to those made above. One of the most effective ways of learning from your practice is to write about it. You will often find that the process of writing about something you did will help to clarify issues for you and focus your ideas. These new insights are often associated with points of real learning about how you practise. Nurses and midwives who practise clinical supervision often spend time writing up the process in their profiles. It is so easy to realise something when discussing a situation you experienced in a supervision session then forget it again in the busy activity of everyday work. Writing about it makes it more likely to be committed to memory, and therefore there is more chance that you will remember it and act accordingly when you come across a similar situation again.

Tool for reflective practice

This has already been discussed on page 5, and will be explored in greater detail in Chapter 6.

Achieving credit as part of a prior learning claim

It is becoming increasingly common for health care professionals to try to gain credit for prior learning and experience when applying to undertake further educational courses. Using the contents of your profile for this purpose needs careful guidance and the ability to recognise what is relevant to your claim and what you should leave out. Some practitioners assume that getting credit for prior learning will be far easier than attending the whole course. This is not the case. We will look at the process of applying for credit in detail in Chapter 7 to give you a realistic idea of what is involved.

Assessment for an educational programme

You may be asked to submit sections of your profile as part of the assessment process for a course or programme you are following. In this case, you need to be quite clear what is expected of you, and the confidentiality of the information you hand in. The confidentiality section of Chapter 6 gives you more information on this.

Lifelong learning

The concept of lifelong learning is widely recognised, not only in health care but also in wider society. The government is keen to encourage people to see learning as something you do throughout your life, and it has set up a number of schemes to help people to get back into learning if they left education some time ago. The Department for Education and Skills has a website specifically looking at lifelong learning (www.lifelonglearning.co.uk), which was set up to help encourage people to take up educational opportunities

Lifelong learning does not just encompass professional knowledge – learning can be undertaken for personal reasons – perhaps you enjoy gardening but want to improve your skills, or would like to learn a language. These are perfectly valid aspects of lifelong learning. However, in health care, developments in knowledge and available treatments and technologies mean it is important for health care professionals to continue to learn throughout their careers. When you gain a professional qualification, you should see it as the first step in an ongoing learning process that will help you to ensure your practice stays up to date. This is the only way you can provide your patients with the high-quality care they need.

The past few years have seen increasing emphasis on the concepts of clinical governance and evidence-based practice in health care. Clinical governance is a process of looking at the way care is delivered and the outcomes for patients. It is undertaken on a national scale by bodies such as the Commission for Health Improvement and the National Institute for

Clinical Excellence, which investigate and report on health care providers and treatments. On a local scale, individual hospitals and trusts monitor their own performance and compare it with previous years and with the performance of other organisations, to give them information on their standards of care.

Evidence-based practice involves using the results of high-quality research and acknowledged best practice to develop and improve practice. In the past, health care delivery tended to develop within individual organisations in particular ways depending on the knowledge, skills, experience and even preferences of individuals within the organisation who had decision-making powers. This is not a systematic way to ensure care is appropriate and based on current knowledge. Health care professionals have been encouraged to change the way they develop care practices and processes, and to ensure they take account of the latest evidence and acknowledged best practice. They are also expected to continue to keep up with developments in their field so that they can adapt their care in the light of new research or practice evidence. These developments mean that, more than ever before, health care employers demand and expect their employees to be flexible, self-motivated and able to transfer skills into new situations with ease, so that they can meet the demands of clinical governance and evidence-based practice. They also expect employees to understand their own strengths and weaknesses, identify their learning needs and ensure they never undertake practices and procedures they are not capable of doing safely. In addition, health care professionals need to demonstrate problem-solving abilities and decision-making skills. This all requires personal confidence and, of course, it requires professionals to be up to date with current knowledge and practice.

There is not enough funding for CPD to enable all health care professionals to meet their learning needs at their employers' expense, while staff shortages can make it difficult to get time off work to attend courses and study days. This means for many health care professionals that the most effective way of meeting most of their learning needs is to do it through their day-to-day practice. By identifying your needs as you go along, and meeting them – by, for example, gaining help, support and advice from colleagues or reading relevant literature – and then putting the learning into practice, you can make your working day a learning opportunity.

The skills involved in developing and maintaining your profile will help you to develop as a lifelong learner. We hope this book will encourage and inspire you to develop a profile that meets your needs, and show you the many ways it can help you meet your professional and personal goals.

REFERENCES

Emap Healthcare Open Learning (1994) *The Profile Pack*, London: EHOL.

English National Board for Nursing, Midwifery and Health Visiting (1991) *ENB Framework for Continuing Professional Education for Nurses, Midwives and Health Visitors: Guide to Implementation*, London: ENB.

English National Board for Nursing, Midwifery and Health Visiting (1995) *Using Your Portfolio: A Resource for Practitioners*, London: ENB.

Nursing and Midwifery Council (2002) *The PREP Handbook*, London: NMC.

Unison (2001) *The HCA Profile: A Personal Development Pack*, London: Unison.

Profiles and Portfolios: The Social Care Context

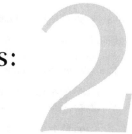

This chapter charts the history and identifies the factors that have influenced the introduction of portfolios into social care.

At any one time around 1.5 million people rely on social services in England, and around 1 million people work in the social care sector. Social Services help and support many of the most vulnerable people in society, and work closely with the National Health Services including the Strategic Health Authorities, NHS Trusts, Care Trusts, the voluntary and private sector and social care organisations. Since the 1998 Government White Paper *Modernising Social Services* (Secretary of State for Health, 1998) the social care agenda has been focused upon modernisation, integrating with the Government White Paper for the NHS – *The NHS Plan* (Department of Health, 2000) and developing and focusing services through representative groups of professional staff and service users.

Modernising Social Services set out its policy for improving social services, including improving standards in the workplace. In outlining why modernisation is needed, the White Paper made clear that its emphasis is on supporting welfare reform and social inclusion by promoting people's independence through providing user-centred services. So, for example, the Long-Term Care Charter has been introduced to make services easier to use and tailored to individual needs. And every council across England is now required to carry out annual satisfaction surveys to monitor the quality of care provision. The government has also set national objectives and priorities for social services for the first time. This means that all councils are required to work to clear standards and consistent rules for how decisions are made on who gets care services.

This agenda has huge implications for staff working in social care. Firstly, staff are now expected to work in partnership with health care services in order to deliver integrated care that is focused on the individual needs of patients/clients. They are also required to work more closely with housing and other services to ensure effective co-ordination of services. Secondly, social care has shifted to a performance culture, and staff are increasingly expected to meet targets for improving the quality and delivery of services provided.

With all this in mind, following on from *Modernising Social Services* the Government set out the first comprehensive national training strategy aimed at analysing the skills needs of people working in the social care sector in England, 'and to develop an action plan to improve the qualification base and the quality of training covered over the coming five years' (*Modernising The Social Care Workforce – The First National Training Strategy For England* (TOPSS, 2000).

The training strategy was agreed and endorsed by Ministers at the Department of Health and Department of Education and Employment in 2000. In addition to the overall training strategy within *Modernising The Social Care Workforce* there is a range of 10 supplementary reports each covering a specific work force group or area of concern as follows:

Residential care (adults) including managers
Child care, including residential care and managers
Learning disability
Mental health
Youth offending team/secure accommodation
Domiciliary care
Drugs and substance misuse
Management development across social care
Registration and inspection
Partnership work, especially with health.

For more information on each of these you can visit the TOPSS website (www.topss.org.uk).

The emphasis in the overall training strategy and supplementary reports is upon:

- improving workforce planning through:
    mapping existing skills and knowledge
    predicting skill and knowledge shortages, gaps and skills mix issues
    recruitment and retention issues
    promotion of best practice
- modernising quality assurance of training outcomes through:
    mapping training against National Occupational and Service Standards

> benchmarking activity
>
> working closely with awarding bodies including higher education institutions

- partnership working:

  > to achieve joint and joined-up services with carers and users to improve training outcomes
  >
  > to ensure employees have the knowledge and skills to work collaboratively
  >
  > to evaluate and monitor all training

(TOPSSEngland, 2000)

The national training strategy also stresses the importance of developing career pathways that support lifelong learning through training and the valuing of personal and professional experience through the Assessment of Prior Experience and Learning (APEL).

The aim of the national training strategy is to develop a culture of lifelong learning so that social care staff are:

- client-centred in their approach
- able to work across traditional professional and service boundaries
- able to build upon their existing knowledge and skills
- able to develop an evidence based approach to their practice and are able to interpret and apply their knowledge.

Evidence-based practice, lifelong learning and portfolio development

Increasingly, social care workers are expected to develop an evidence-based approach to their practice. Evidence-based practice means placing the clients' benefits first. Evidence-based practitioners adopt a process of lifelong learning that involves continually posing specific questions of direct practical importance to clients, searching objectively and efficiently for the best evidence relative to each question and taking appropriate action guided by evidence. Gibbs (2002) offers useful support on this subject.

Becoming a lifelong learner is essential to becoming an evidence-based practitioner. This is because being a lifelong learner involves continuously thinking about, updating and maintaining your professional knowledge and skills.

At its simplest, profiling helps you to become a lifelong learner. It is a structured approach to helping you to identify what your already know and can do, identify weaknesses that you would like to address and an action plan for achieving your goals.

Standards for social care

The General Social Care Council

The General Social Care Council (GSCC) is a non-departmental government body that works closely with the Department of Health. It was established in 2001 under the Care Standards Act 2000, and its job is to regulate the social care workforce and to promote high standards of care within the social care sector.

In September 2002 the GSCC introduced the first codes of practice for social care workers and employers. These codes set out the standards of practice and conduct social care workers and their employers are expected to meet. The GSCC is also tasked with regulating and supporting social work education and training. So, for example, it is responsible for accrediting universities offering social work qualifications and approved courses.

In 2003, the GSCC launched the Social Care Register, which means that all social care workers in England must now be registered practitioners. In short, to register you must hold an appropriate qualification and commit to upholding the Codes of Practice for Social Care Workers, and be physically fit to do your job.

The Codes of Practice for social workers set out the standards of social care practice and the conduct workers and employers are expected to meet. The code has been developed largely by social care workers, service users and carers themselves. It aims to build on good practice and shared values within the social care sector. The code means that, for the first time, social care workers will, like nurses and doctors be registered. And, in common with nurses and doctors, breaching the code could mean being removed from the register.

The code of practice for social care workers is enforced by employers.

Occupational standards for social care

The National Occupational Standards for Social Care (NOS) were approved by the Qualifications and Curriculum Authority in 2002. The standards reflect the minimum standards of practice required, and are relevant to the competence of a beginner social worker. The standards also support the principles of lifelong learning.

The development of strategies for supporting lifelong learning are seen as essential to delivering *The NHS Plan* and *Modernising Social Services*. The national document *Working Together – Learning Together: A Framework*

For Lifelong Learning In The NHS (Department of Health, 2001) sets out a framework for lifelong learning in health and social care. Put simply, this paper recognises that the strategies of lifelong learning will enable staff to improve the services and care they provide, and are crucial to addressing organisational and cultural change. *Working Together – Learning Together* sets out a comprehensive action plan, covering the period up to 2005, for how this will be achieved. In particular it makes the following clear statements that individual practitioners should:

• seek opportunities to participate in personal learning and development and to influence and shape team and/or organisational strategies for lifelong learning
• agree a personal development with their line manager which identifies and addresses their learning needs, links with key skills and organisational goals and lifelong learning and supports improvements in patient care and services
• take responsibility where appropriate, for supporting the learning and development needs of others.

Developing a personal profile is one way of supporting social care staff in achieving these goals. In particular a profile will help you to:

• identify how you learn best, where you learn best and your strengths and weaknesses
• identify how you can contribute to a culture of lifelong learning within your organisation both on an individual level as well as within the team
• help you to assess how you can support the lifelong learning needs of colleagues including peers as well as those for whom you might have responsibility
• develop a goal and action plan to help you to achieve these goals.

The starting point for the development of the occupational standards was a definition of the key purpose of social work – for which the international definition of social work was adopted as follows:

A profession which promotes social change, problem-solving in human relationships, and the empowerment and liberation of people to enhance well-being. Utilising theories of human behaviour, and social systems, social work intervenes at the points where people interact with their environments. Principles of human rights and social justice are fundamental to social work.
(International Federation of Social Workers, 2000)

The occupational standards, therefore, recognise and support the holistic nature of social care, and, as with health care, recognise the importance of an agreed code of professional values and ethics for competent social care practice.

Continuing professional development

Social care workers who hold a recognised professional social work qualification are eligible to study for a post-qualifying award. Post Qualifying Training means that social care workers can continue their professional development beyond their initial qualification through studying one of six post-qualifying awards:

Post Qualifying Award in Social Work
Advanced Award in Social Work
Mental Health Social Work Award
Child Care Award
Practice Teaching Award
Regulation of Care Services Award

Currently post-qualifying development is not a requirement of registration. However, in the future social care practitioners, in line with their colleagues in health care, will be expected to show evidence of ongoing learning and development as a requirement for re-registration.

As there is little or no funding available to support continuing professional development, it is likely that social care staff will be expected to update their practice through their own initiatives, and not necessarily through attending a taught course or formal training. Rather, like health care practioners, social care workers will be expected to update their practice through:

- attending conferences
- reading professional journals
- attending informal training events offered through local or regional networks

In particular, social care staff – whether registered for a formal qualification or simply updating their practice for re-registration – will be encouraged to link their learning to the UK occupational standards, which have been developed and agreed by the national training organisation, TOPSS. The existing post-qualifying framework was introduced by the Central Council

For Education and Training In Social Work (CCETSW) in 1990. One of the key features of the post-qualifying framework was the introduction of a credit accumulation scheme (CATS) (for a clear description of CATS see page 106). The beauty of this scheme is that it recognises that people learn in different ways – and not simply through attending a course or lecture. Because of the changes in social care, especially with regulation of the workforce, together with changes in the size, structure and nature of the roles undertaken by staff, the current post-qualifying framework is under review.

REFERENCES

Department of Health (2000) *The NHS Plan: A Plan for Investment, a Plan for Reform.* London: The Stationery Office.

Department of Health (2001) *Working Together, Learning Together: A Framework for Lifelong Learning for the NHS.* London: The Stationery Office.

Gibbs, L. (2002) *Evidence-based Practice for the Helping Professions: A Practical Guide with Integrated Multimedia.* Belmont, CA: Brooks Cole.

International Federation of Social Workers (2000) *Definition of Social Work.* www.ifsw.org.

Secretary of State for Health (1998) *Modernising Social Services: Promoting Independence, Improving Protection Raising Standards.* London: The Stationery Office.

Training Organisation for the Personal Social Services (2000) *Modernising the Social Care Workforce: The First National Training Strategy for England.* Leeds: TOPSS England.

Getting to Grips with the Terminology

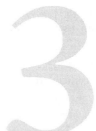

The introduction of the profile has brought with it a new range of jargon that is unfamiliar and at times confusing. To make matters worse, the terms profile and portfolio are often used interchangeably and sometimes inaccurately. This chapter attempts to explain the terminology and unravel the jargon by clarifying the following terms: continuing professional development, lifelong learning, profile, portfolio, experiential learning, reflection, learning outcomes, APL and APEL.

The introduction of profiles into health and social care has brought with it new terms and jargon with which you may not be familiar. Some of these terms, such as 'lifelong learning', are used within government policies as well as within health and social care practice. Many terms come from the context of adult, further and higher education and, whilst not difficult to understand, can be unfamiliar. This chapter will help you to understand the distinctions and meanings behind some of the key terms associated with profiles. It should help you understand what people are talking about when they use the terms and enable you to use them accurately within your own professional language. All the terms described here will also be considered in more depth in the other chapters.

Lifelong learning

Learning is the key to prosperity – for each of us as individuals, as well as for the nation as a whole. Learning throughout life will build human capital by encouraging the acquisition of knowledge and skills and emphasising creativity and imagination. The fostering of an enquiring mind and the love of learning are essential to our future success. (David Blunkett, Secretary of State for Education and Employment, 1998)

In 1998, the government introduced its Green Paper *The Learning Age* (Department for Education and Employment, 1998). In this paper it set out its vision of the learning age in which 'the development of a culture of learning will help to build a united society' and support individuals to become more independent. Within this vision lifelong learning is seen as essential to both a strong economy and an inclusive society by offering a way 'out of dependency and low expectation'. Since the Green Paper the government has introduced a number of policies and initiatives to support the development of lifelong learning. To read more about these you can access the lifelong learning website: www.lifelonglearning.co.uk.

Briefly, however, within the context of health and social care, learning and development is seen as the key to delivering patient/client-centred care. This is because lifelong learning is not just about acquiring new skills. It is also about supporting you to build upon what you already know and can do so as to change and improve your own practice and enhance the care you provide.

Lifelong learning and work

In 2000, *The NHS Plan* set out the government's plans for improving the education, training and professional development of health and social care staff. Subsequently, in 2001, it set out its core vision for implementing these plans in *Working Together – Learning Together: A Framework for Lifelong Learning* (Department of Health, 2001).

In chapter 1 of *Working Together, Learning Together, Lifelong Learning: The Context – Core Values and Skills*, the government makes a strong argument for the important contribution lifelong learning makes in improving patient/client care. This document states reasons why it is important that you continue to grow and develop as a professional including:

- Changes to the wider world of work, the diversity of people's lifestyles and cultures and their changing expectations about work and learning
- Changing patterns of healthcare delivery
- The opportunities offered by new technologies to harness and share knowledge and know-how through increasing access to learning in the workplace
- Advances in health technologies and interventions, increased availability of research-based knowledge, the rise of empowered, knowledgeable consumers and their increasing expectations of the care they receive
- Continuing shifts in the boundaries between primary, secondary and

continuing care combined with new ways of delivering care, new standards for care and the reshaping of processes and pathways to support care that is patient/client-centred.
- A more diverse workforce entering careers from a wider variety of backgrounds, cultures and ages, with differing learning and development styles and needs
- A greater emphasis on team working and on developing partnership working between organisations and practitioners to deliver care for whole communities.

At the heart of this vision lies the belief that professional development should be valued by everyone working in the NHS and that learning programmes should be based on individual needs and rooted in practice as follows:

- Access to education, training and development should be as open and flexible as possible – with no discrimination in terms of age, gender, ethnicity, availability to part-time and full-time staff, geographical locations
- Learning should be valued, recognised, recorded and accredited wherever possible
- Wherever practical, learning should be shared by different staff groups and professions.

In addition, all health and social care staff should:

- fully understand and respect the rights and feelings of patients/clients and their families, seeking out and addressing their needs
- communicate effectively with patients/clients, their families and carers and their colleagues
- work effectively in teams, appreciating the roles of other staff and agencies involved in care
- demonstrate a commitment to keeping their skills and competence up to date – including the use of new approaches to learning and using information, and supporting the learning and development of others.
(Department of Health, 2001)

Increasingly, then we are being encouraged to learn all the time in formal and informal ways; through study, as well as through watching television, taking an evening class and from family and friends.

The belief that learning happens throughout our lives and is lifelong is fundamental to the concept of profiling. Most of us have acquired knowledge and skills as we have gone through life that we either do not recognise we possess or underutilise. Profiling, therefore, is a process that will help you to identify some of the knowledge and skills you possess and present them in a way that can be recognised by yourself and others. It is worth remembering that learning does not always have a 'sell by' date on it. Some of the learning we acquired a long time ago can still be utilised today, whilst more current learning might prove to be out of date or redundant.

Continuing professional development (CPD)

Continuing professional development, then, refers to any lifelong learning activities you undertake once you have qualified. (Although if you are seeking accreditation for prior learning you might identify learning that you have gained before you registered. See page 102.) As we have said, continuing to develop your practice once you have qualified will keep you up to date with new developments in knowledge, understanding, technical skills and procedures. Just as the professions are constantly changing, so also you as a practitioner need to be able to adapt to the changes and to prepare yourself for additional roles that may be demanded of you. In short, health and social care practitioners need to be far more self-aware and reflective in their practice.

The rapidly changing scene of the health and social services in the early years of the new millennium means that you need to be adaptable, flexible and able to expand your expertise and practice in response to what is happening around you. This is at the heart of lifelong learning and the need for CPD. It not only means getting to grips with a new knowledge base because of some new type of treatment that is now available, but also includes understanding the skills you possess and how they can be transferred from one situation to another. In 1994 the English National Board for Nursing and Midwifery described lifelong learning in ways which are relevant to the context of current health and social care. According to this description lifelong learners are:

- **innovative** in their practice
- **flexible** to changing demand
- **resourceful** in their methods of working
- able to work as **change agents**
- able to **share good practice** and knowledge
- **adaptable** to changing health care needs
- **challenging** and **creative** in their practice
- **self-reliant** in their way of working
- **responsible and accountable** for their actions

It is our belief that one of the best ways to achieve these characteristics is through developing a profile approach to learning. This is because in today's health and social care environment it is extremely likely that you will be expected to achieve these characteristics through your own learning initiative and not from attending a continuing education programme.

In addition, if you are to develop as a practitioner you will also have to develop as a person. Although personal and professional development are sometimes expressed as separate activities, in reality they are one and the same thing. Unless you lead two very different lives that begin and end at your front door, it is very difficult to prevent things you learn from your private life experience spilling over into your working life, and vice versa. It is only relatively recently, and because of the increasing use of profiles, that we have realised the benefits of not making false divisions between personal and professional life. It is also true that health and social care workers represent around 90 per cent of the overall workforce in the health service (including the public and private sectors). This force of numbers means that you are the most important resource in making sure the service achieves its purpose. It also means that if you do not develop, the service will not develop.

In 1999, the Government introduced *Continuing Professional Development: Quality in the NHS* (Department of Health, 1999), which sets out its plans for supporting lifelong learning initiatives and continuing professional development for all NHS staff. In this it argues that the long-term vision for CPD is based on the core principles that it should be:

- purposeful and patient/client-centred
- participative; i.e. fully involving the individual and other relevant stakeholders, targeted at identical educational need, educationally effective
- part of a wider organisational development plan in support of local and national service objectives
- focused on the development needs of teams, across traditional professional and service boundaries
- designed to build on previous knowledge, skills and experience
- designed to enhance the skills of interpreting and applying knowledge based on research and development.

The Government has introduced a number of initiatives to support lifelong learning and continuing professional development. These include:

Cadet schemes These schemes combine work experience with theoretical learning, leading typically to an NVQ in Care at level 3.
NHS learning accounts (LAs) *The NHS Plan* published in July 2000

said that over the following three years NHS staff who did not have a professional qualification would have access to either an NHS LA of up to £150 or dedicated training and assessment to NVQ levels 2 and 3.

Modern Apprenticeships (MAs)   These are a mix of work-based training and education that include an NVQ, key skills and a technical certificate.

Basic Skills   The Skills for Life Strategy has allocated funds to improve literacy and numeracy skills.

Foundation Degrees   These offer a two-year vocational degree worth at least 240 credits that will be delivered flexibly including part-time or through distance learning so that you can continue to learn at work.

For more information on any of these initiatives as well as others see www.doh.gov.uk/lifelonglearning

Profiles and portfolios

As we have said, profiles and portfolios are terms that are often used interchangeably. The producers of profiles and portfolios have added to the problems by selling products that essentially look the same, whilst calling them different names. It is difficult to know why and how this differing use of the terms has arisen, and to some extent it does not matter. Having identified that confusion exists, this alerts you to the fact that it is important to find out how someone is using the term so that you are able to share their perceptions before jumping to conclusions.

The way the terms are used often comes from the particular purpose of the profile or portfolio. For example, the term most frequently associated with the accreditation of prior experiential learning (APEL) is portfolio preparation. Most people if asked what a portfolio is, would probably think of an art portfolio. Indeed, Brown (1995) has argued that an art portfolio influenced her definition of a portfolio:

> An art portfolio is a private collection of evidence which demonstrates the continuing acquisition of skills, knowledge, attitudes and achievements. It is both retrospective and prospective, as well as reflecting the current state of development and activity of the individual.

Thinking of your portfolio as an art portfolio is not a bad idea. An art portfolio is simply a collection of material that aims to demonstrate the owner's artistic development. It can include drawings, writing or sculpture. It can be big or small; it can be thick; it can be thin. Ideally it is not judged in terms of volume, but rather by its relevance and quality. All of this is very close to how a portfolio is used. Indeed, to show how varied your profile might be Brown has produced the diagram shown here in Figure 3.1:

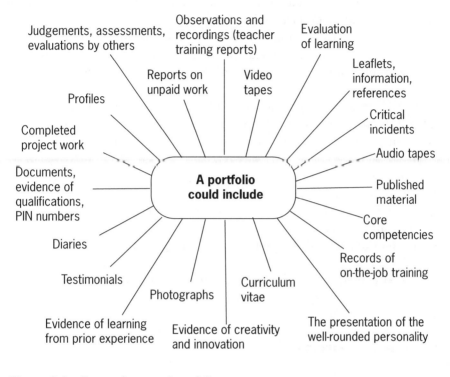

Figure 3.1   Types of personal portfolio
Source: R. Brown (1995) in Clark, E. and Rogers, J. (eds) *Developing your Professional Portfolio*

So, a portfolio of prior learning is simply a record of your past learning and learning achievements. It does not have to be written and it can contain drawings, a computer package, a video or even a sculpture. Indeed, the majority of guidelines for constructing a portfolio do not seek to prescribe what should be included or how it should be presented. Most often the guidelines state that the portfolio should enable you to keep a record of your personal and professional development, your professional experiences and qualifications. It is seen as a way for you to develop skills of critical reflective practice, to consider experiences in your professional and personal life and to evaluate the contribution these experience make to your development and to improvements in client/patient care.

Profiling has sometimes been chosen because the development team feel that the word most accurately portrays the personal development aspects of profile work. From this perspective, profiling is important to you for two reasons:

- As an individual: understanding and appreciating the significance of what and how you learn involves an ongoing process of reflection that will enhance your self-awareness and build confidence in the value of your life and experience to date
- As a professional: having an effective and up-to-date record of your past and current learning and experience will provide you with a powerful means of communication with employers, both present and future.

In this approach, a professional profile is expected to acknowledge the integrity or wholeness of the individual. Generally speaking these are characteristics that are common to a profile and a portfolio. They both:

- value experience as a source of learning
- encourage reflective practice
- provide a storehouse for information about and evidence of experience, learning and achievements
- encourage personal and professional development.

As stated earlier, we will be using the term 'profile' throughout the book, unless referring to a specific product called a portfolio.

Experiential learning

Whilst experiential learning is often very much part of the assessment of learning, its meanings and traditions have a far broader application. To get to grips with what profiling is all about, it is useful to understand what experiential learning means and its relevance to this context. People learn from a wide variety of sources. They learn from relationships with friends, family and colleagues. They learn from social activities such as sport, voluntary work, travel and reading – in fact, from every activity in which they are involved. However, although people clearly learn from experience, not all experiences lead to learning.

The starting point in discussing what we mean by experiential learning, therefore, is to ask how experience is related to learning. Experiential educators have had many arguments over this question. Nevertheless, nearly all would agree with John Dewey, an American philosopher generally regarded as one of the early key figures in experiential education. Dewey (1933) argues that for experience to become learning it needs to include 'an active and passive element peculiarly combined. On the active hand, experience is trying . . . On the passive it is undergoing'. In other words, for Dewey, learning from experience is making 'backward and forward connections between what we do to things and what we enjoy or suffer from things as a consequence'.

So in experiential learning the learner is directly involved with the realities being studied. This can be contrasted with learning which is only read, heard, talked or written about, but where the reality of practice is never brought into the process.

In more recent times the work of David Kolb (1984) has elucidated the basic principles of experiential learning. Influenced by philosophers such as Dewey, Kolb argues for a relationship between thinking and experience. He views experiential learning as a cycle involving action and reflection, theory and practice. When profiles are used primarily as a learning *tool* they tend to adopt the framework of Kolb's learning cycle. We shall therefore be returning to explore Kolb's work in greater depth elsewhere.

So far we have said that experiential learning involves not merely theory but practice, not simply observing but doing. This is one of the reasons why it is seen as a particularly effective approach to continuing professional development. As a tool in professional development, experiential learning is certainly not new. Rather, we can see it reflected in the craft guilds and apprenticeship systems that provided so much advanced training from the mediaeval period through to the industrial revolution. Then, as now, people learnt experientially and informally, whilst at the same time having more formal systems of education provided by monks and clergy in monasteries and churches. So, in one sense there is nothing startling or revelatory about experiential learning. It is simply that academic and professional education is increasingly recognising its benefits and is therefore seeking to foster approaches to education that build upon learning from and through experience.

Another aspect of experiential learning is the emphasis placed upon links between affective and cognitive learning. If people really do gain so much quality learning from their life and social situations, they have to acknowledge the importance of their emotions in this process. So, for example, learning is often acquired through highly emotional experiences such as bereavement, falling in love, and divorce. Traditionally, affective learning has been disregarded because it appears to be a subjective activity, difficult to assess within formal education. However, as we shall be emphasising throughout this book, affective learning is, in theory, no more difficult to assess than cognitive learning (which is concerned with factual knowledge, comprehension and application).

If personal experiences are genuinely regarded as the substance of learning, then the distinctive boundaries created between academic and professional disciplines become more nonsensical and need to be dismantled. It does not make sense to ask learners to experience academically one minute and practically the next, or to think historically in one learning situation and mathematically or medically in the next.

As you can see, experiential learning can therefore refer simply to a technique of developing practice-based education, or it can be associated with a whole philosophy of education that supports the notion of open, learner-centred learning. Many experiential educators see experiential learning as:

> A means by which we cease to fragment our experience and our ways of knowing: for instance, intellectual, intuitive, social and behavioural. Through experiential learning cycles and processes, we learn to see underlying patterns and connections, and powerful central themes within larger wholes. Making sense of ourselves in relation to the world is at the centre of experiential learning. (Weil and McGill, 1989)

Experiential learning is central to everything you do in health and social care. It is important in informing the decisions you make and the support you offer clients and patients.

Reflection

Because reflection is at the heart of profiling we have dedicated a chapter to exploring the theory of reflective practice (see Chapter 6). However, in the current chapter we simply provide you with a brief overview of what it is. All approaches to experiential learning view action and reflection as the basis for learning. In this sense reflection is taken to mean a collection of activities, which might include simply sitting in a corner mulling over thoughts. It can also be a much more dynamic process that involves writing, discussion and learning from conversations with colleagues and friends.

Reflection is now recognised as an essential component of professional practice, one of the early pioneers of reflective practice was Donald Schon, particularly since the publication of his first book *The Reflective Practitioner* (1983) which looked at the different ways in which we act and reflect in and on action. Schon challenged the traditional assumption that professional practice is simply the application of a task or a display of relevant knowledge to clearly defined problems. We discuss his ideas more fully in Chapter 6. However, it is worth noting that it is Schon's view of professional practice that is at the heart of evidence-based practice. Because evidence-based practice is simply the process by which you make decisions using the best available evidence, your expertise and client/patient choice.

Reflection in the context of learning suggests that reflective practitioners are:

Conducting a conversation. The conversation has a critical edge to it, for the professional is always asking the question: what if . . . ? Being faced with fresh problems to which there is no single answer, and no one right answer, the professional has the responsibility to appraise the situation and formulate an effective strategy. The effective professional, has, accordingly, to be continually self-critical. (Barnett, 1992)

Reflection, then is at the heart of health and social care practice as you continually make connections between what you already know, what members of your team know, external evidence and what your client/patient wants.

In the context of profiling, the concept of reflective practice therefore has two important elements. First and foremost reflection is regarded as an activity that can occur at any time after experience. Indeed, reflection is viewed as an active process that turns the experience into learning. An Australian educator, David Boud has written extensively on the role of reflection in learning. Boud *et al.* (1985) take the view that most people are largely unaware of their internal processes for learning. However, once they become aware and skilled at using them, they are likely to become much more effective practitioners. For Boud, reflection is simply a generic term for the mental activities people carry out in order for learning to occur. Because of the importance of reflection and action in the development of any approach to the profile process, we look at this in much greater depth in Chapter 6 (Profiles and Reflective Practice).

Learning outcomes

The increasing use of learning outcomes has been one way in which a variety of professions, and accrediting bodies have sought to create a balance between giving recognition to what people can do and allowing them to develop their own private record of ongoing personal development. At their simplest, learning outcomes are a clearly worked out description of what people need to demonstrate they have achieved in order to have their learning assessed, usually against a particular qualification or award. Learning outcomes are also used by course developers to show the intention of the programme. For example, each module within a programme will have a set of learning outcomes that need to be achieved. This is helpful when you are going to use evidence from your profile to show which parts of the programme you do not need to repeat. Another way in which learning outcomes are used is to make clear to learners what they are being assessed against, but to do so in a way that does not prescribe what should be included and allows them to demonstrate particular qualities and knowledge as well as skills from their own experience. Some portfolios have been designed to reflect characteristics that represent areas of skill, knowledge and expertise health care workers must have in order to provide the quality of care required to meet the changing health care needs of the public.

Multidisciplinary teams: the challenge for CPD

Increasingly, you will work in a multidisciplinary team that might cross primary, community and acute sectors of care. You might already be working in a multidisciplinary setting. Whether this is the case or not, it is important that where possible you take the opportunity for shared learning across traditional boundaries of health and social care. This does not mean that you will lose your specialist knowledge. Multidisciplinary team working means working with others to build a culture of shared values and understanding between different groups of practitioners. You might want to explore the ways in which you work in multidisciplinary ways in your profile.

Progress files and personal development planning (HE)

In 1997, the National Committee of Inquiry into Higher Education recommended that higher education institutions should improve the quality and consistency of information on the learning and achievement of students in higher education by introducing progress files. Progress files consist of two elements. Firstly, they provide a record of an individual's learning and achievement by the institution. Secondly, they provide individual learners with a personal record of learning and achievements, including progress reviews and plans and goal and action planning for their own personal educational and career development. Personal development planning is the term used to describe this process.

Higher education institutions have developed individual approaches to personal development planning. However, the process involved shares similar characteristics to that involved in producing a profile or portfolio. In particular, personal development planning is structured to help individuals to reflect upon their own learning, performance and achievement and to plan personal career and educational goals. For further information on personal development planning: www.qaa.ac.uk

Credit frameworks

In November 2002 the Qualifications and Curriculum Authority (QCA) and the National Learning and Skills Council (LSC) made recommendations to the government on the role of credit in relation to learning and skills and the development of a National Qualification Framework. As a result, in January 2003 the LSC was asked to establish a working group to develop national principles for credit practice, specifications, and terminology and QA systems. The development of credit frameworks means that the higher and further education sectors have developed an approach to credit that has many applications. Essential features of National Qualifications Framework are that it:

- provides a single framework encompassing all post-16 achievement from entry level to postgraduate/professional level
- adopts a common language for describing achievement and in particular clarity about the distinction between units of assessment and delivery
- describes and measures all achievement, whether vocational, general or academic in the same way.

All sorts of national qualifications exist within the National Qualifications Framework, which is broken into three categories and six levels (entry level to level 5). This means that the National Qualifications Framework aims to:

- avoid duplication and overlap of qualifications – so that you don't have to re-learn what you already know and can do
- provide clear progression routes for students – so that you can continue to learn and develop throughout your life.

For further information about credit frameworks: www.lsda.org.uk and www.qca.org.uk

Key skills

Key skills are those that are commonly needed to be successful in education, work and life. These key skills are:

application of numbers (numeracy)
communication
improving own learning and performance
information technology

problem solving
working with others.

For more information on key skills: *www.qca.org.uk*

Glossary of terms

Accreditation of prior experiential learning (APEL) This is the process through which you can obtain academic credit for informal learning you have gained through work, home and social life.

Accreditation of prior learning (APL) This is the process whereby you can get credit for learning you have gained through formal study, such as a attending a course which has not already been recognised.

========================= **REFERENCES** =========================

Barnett, R. (1992) *Learning to Effect,* London: SRHE/OU.

Boud, D., Keogh, R., Walker, D. (1985) *Reflection: Turning Experiences into Learning,* London: Kogan Page.

Brown, R. (1995) *Portfolio Development and Profiling for Nurses* (2nd edn), Lancaster, Central Health Studies, in Clark, E. and Rogers, J. (1996) *Developing Your Professional Portfolio,* Edinburgh: Churchill Livingstone.

Department for Education and Employment (1998) *The Learning Age: A New Renaissance for a New Britain,* London: The Stationery Office.

Department of Health (1999) *Continuing Professional Development: Quality in the New NHS,* London: The Stationery Office.

Department of Health (2000) *The NHS Plan: A Plan for Investment, a Plan for Reform,* London: The Stationery Office.

Department of Health (2001) *Working Together, Learning Together: A Framework for Lifelong Learning for the NHS,* London: The Stationery Office

Dewey, J. (1933) *How We Think,* Boston, MA: DC Heath.

Kolb, D. (1984) *Experiential Learning: Experience as a Source of Learning and Development,* New Jersey: Prentice Hall.

Schon, D. (1984) *The Reflective Practitioner,* New York: Basic Books.

Weil, S., and McGill, I. (eds) (1989) *Making Sense of Experiential Learning,* London: SRHE/OU Press.

Some Common Themes and Questions Shared

This chapter will help you to think about what you need to begin developing your profile. We explore the 10 most common questions people ask, including:

- Why do I need to compile a profile?
- Should I buy a ready-made profile?
- How do I decide which profile to buy?
- How long will it take to complete?

When you begin developing your profile, it usually feels like uncharted territory. Being asked to reflect upon your life experience feels endless and overwhelming. These are some of the most common comments made:

- 'I am 48. I've been around for a long time. That's a lot of experience to think about. I don't know where to start.'
- 'I haven't done anything significant. I haven't any experiences worth reflecting on.'
- 'It feels frightening. I am worried it is going to throw up feelings I would rather forget.'
- 'I don't know what it is you are looking for.'
- 'It's wonderful. I've not stopped thinking about myself all week.'
- 'I didn't realise I had done so much. I didn't realise I had so much to offer.'
- 'What has been surprising to me is how interesting it is. I've never really thought about what I have done before or how I feel.'
  (Comments made by students attending profile classes, Goldsmiths College, University of London, 1992)

For some people the process can seem daunting because they have lived and learnt so much; whereas some are lost because they feel they have not lived or learnt at all. They might feel excited by thinking about their experiences, often for the first time; but by opening themselves up in this way, they also fear they could expose themselves to feelings and emotions that they would rather forget, or that will leave them feeling vulnerable. In addition, whilst feeling good about recognising the extent of their own experience and learning, some people feel unsure about what an assessing panel or awarding body is looking for and whether the learning they identify is relevant or at an appropriate standard.

In the next chapter we explore some of these issues and offer practical suggestions as to how you might work effectively through the profile process. Because each profile is unique, each person will approach its construction in a different way. This, in turn, means that each person will have unique issues and questions that they need to address as they begin work. To help you to identify some of these issues, therefore, this chapter explores the 10 most common questions initially asked about profiling. Within each of these you will wish to identify a subset of questions and issues of your own. You will find that there are few right or wrong answers. Rather, you will need to think about how you work best and decide which is the right answer for you. The views expressed here are those held by the authors – be prepared to question what is being said, and to contribute a few ideas of your own.

Why do I need to compile a profile?

Throughout this book we stress that profiling provides a flexible approach to professional development, offering people greater choice over what they want to learn and how they want to develop as health or social care professionals. However, many practitioners argue that profiling actually limits choice, as it is, for some, now a compulsory element of professional development. Since 1995 all nurses, health visitors and midwives have been required to complete a profile in order to register. It is true that by making profiling a compulsory component of registration, nurses and midwives have little choice as to whether or not to complete it. However, the profile process itself is far from limiting. Rather, it enhances and broadens your opportunities and maximises your personal and professional potential.

It is important to bear in mind that, as a professional, you are responsible for maintaining the effectiveness of your practice. Ideas about the profession in which you are working change continually. As a professional you need to be aware of these ideas and how they impinge on your everyday practices. Within this context, profiling offers maximum choice about what you want to learn and how you want to develop in the future. Profiling, therefore, provides the most appropriate method for addressing professional development needs.

The best profile is one that *supports* your professional development in a number of ways. In particular, it will enable you to develop the skills to reflect upon and assess critically what you know and can do. Once you are able to articulate the range and depth of your learning, both to yourself and to others, you are in a much stronger position to be able to make decisions about courses you wish to attend and the knowledge you want to develop in the future. So, profiling enables you to identify realistic and relevant future educational goals.

Should I buy a ready-made profile?

There are two main reasons why people buy a ready-made profile. The first is that some profiles have been 'tailor made' for a specific purpose and to match a specific set of prescribed learning outcomes. The second is that buying a profile offers a ready-made structure in a professionally designed format.

However, you should not feel obliged to buy a profile off the shelf. Many people can and do create their own well-organised and professional profile. Indeed, some organisations regard the skills required in the personal design of a profile as an integral part of the learning process, and it is sometimes possible to gain accreditation for this additional effort. Developing a profile from scratch simply takes a little more planning at the outset.

How do I decide which profile to buy?

There are a number of profiles on the market and it is worthwhile investing time in deciding which one is best for you.

Deciding which profile to buy requires the same approach as for choosing any major product. Begin by clarifying your aims and establishing criteria before deciding which is the most appropriate. This will combine common sense and personal preference. For example, when deciding which car to buy, your decisions will be based upon how much driving you do (comfort, cost of petrol, etc.), your garage/car space, the image you want to project, maintenance cost, and personal colour preference. When deciding which profile to buy, the areas you need to consider are purpose, accessibility, content, design and layout, and cost.

Purpose

Whether you are buying a profile off the shelf or building your own, the first step is to clarify with whom you are seeking to communicate. If, for example, you are seeking to use your profile to apply for a particular job, you will be communicating with colleagues, usually at a more senior level, working in the same profession. If, by contrast, you wish to submit your profile for academic purposes, you will be communicating with academic staff who might be new to your profession and its language. So, whatever your purpose, when embarking on a profile you need to consider how it will be received and, above all, by whom.

Having said this, most people will be developing a profile for two reasons: firstly, to enhance professional development in the broadest terms; secondly, for a range of purposes which might include applying for jobs, access to academic credit, and/or retaining professional registration.

Whatever your purpose, it is important to remember that the profile is a process which enables you to communicate more effectively with yourself and others. The best profile, therefore, is one which provides you with both a private and public record.

A private record: communicating with yourself

Profiling is a system of discovering and recording information about your personal and professional life. Some of the information you choose to include in the profile, therefore, will be sensitive and you will want it to remain private. Through the private record you may also wish to experiment with developing a writing style, or with new ideas and concepts. In addition, you may wish to decide to share your private record with a few, carefully selected people. A good profile, therefore, enables you to record your thoughts privately – perhaps in a way that will only make sense to yourself.

A public record: communicating with others

The vast majority of what you include in the profile will be public. You need to ensure, therefore, that the information you include is easy to read, accessible and well organised.

You will almost certainly wish to include a section about your past employment, education, training and qualifications, as well as biographical details. This might sound like an enhanced curriculum vitae and, in some respects, this is certainly true. However, your professional profile is not simply a record of what you have done; it is also an important record of your personal skills and abilities. Recording these should help you to identify strengths that you did not know you possessed, together with areas you would like to develop and improve. In short, the profile is expected to demonstrate your 'ongoing' professional development. Some profiles have sections and exercises to assist you with this, including the identification of goals and action plans for the future. Others, by contrast, simply refer to a bibliography of suggested reading.

Accessibility

It is essential that the material in the profile you purchase is accessible and has relevance for you. When buying one, you should consider the following:

- Is it written clearly and in a language I can understand?
- Are any difficult terms or concepts clearly explained?
- Is it versatile? Are each of the sections independent of each other, allowing me to move around easily within the material as a whole?
- Are there any guidelines on how to use the materials?
- Are there activities or materials which enable me to reflect upon and evaluate my past as well as current learning?

Content

The reason most people find difficulty in deciding which profile to buy is that they have no clear idea what they want to use it for – they simply know they have to complete one. Once you know what kind of profile you wish to produce, you will find it easier to choose a profile that is best suited to meeting your needs.

In deciding which profile to buy, however, it is important that you do not opt for the one which appears to provide the softest option, offering very few challenges. Working through exercises which enable you to understand the depth and range of your knowledge is a crucial part of the process. Constructing a profile is not always easy, and is rarely straightforward. Most people who have completed a profile say it is both demanding and time-consuming. They also say that it is well worth the effort and extremely rewarding:

> I found reflecting on my personal life much harder than I had thought it would be. Some of the skills I have learned go as far back in my child-hood to when I worked in an old people's home as a Saturday helper. When I began to reflect it felt like an enormous task. Now, I can see it is a skill I've developed. I find it easier to make connections with my past experiences now. In fact I find it exciting to learn more and more about what makes me tick. I can now see the fruits of my labour. I want to continue developing my portfolio forever! (Hull, 1993)

So, when deciding which profile to buy, ask yourself:

- Will this profile challenge me to think?
- Will it enable me to learn more about myself and to make connections with my past and current learning?
- Will it integrate my personal and professional learning?
- Is the content flexible enough for me to use it for a variety of purposes?
- Will I be able to develop my portfolio rapidly and with ease?

Design and layout

The design and layout are important factors to consider, both in terms of presentation and ease of use.

Binder

A profile binder must be sturdy enough to withstand heavy use as you continually put things into it, take things out and move material around within it. In choosing a binder, therefore, consider the following:

- How strong is it: will it stand up to perpetual use?
- Is it the right size in depth and length?
- Does it present the appropriate image?
- Can you carry it around or will it be too bulky?

Dividers

- Will they withstand perpetual use?
- Are they easy to differentiate? (Remember: your profile will eventually be filled with paper.)

Forms

Some profiles provide forms for you to include in your finished document.

- Are they clear and easy to use?
- Are they appropriate (both in level and content)?
- Can they be photocopied easily?
- Can you obtain more copies if necessary?
- Do they look professional?

Workbooks

Some profiles include workbooks and materials.

- Is the language clear and accessible?

- Is the spine strong, or will it crack with perpetual use?
- Will it be easy to use?

Considering the layout is also important.

- Is it attractive and appealing?
- Does it interest you?
- Will you be able to move around the materials easily and can you open the workbook at any point and begin?

General content

- Is there a glossary of terms to help you understand any jargon?
- Is there a bibliography of further reading?
- Are there activities and materials to stimulate your thinking?
- Will any of the information given help you in constructing the profile?
- Are there materials to help you develop your writing skills?
- Does it include a professional record of your formal learning and qualifications?
- How much room is there to include details of your informal, personal and 'on-the-job' learning?
- Is there information on where to go if you need further help?

Cost

Clearly, cost is an important consideration. As with buying any product, the most expensive profile might not necessarily be the best one. Deciding how much to spend will largely be determined by how much you can afford and which profile best fulfils your criteria.

What can I put into it?

Most people know and can do far more than they think they can. In particular, they barely recognise the extent to which their informal, experiential learning is used in professional practice. This is largely because learning in our culture is so frequently associated with formal qualifications that uncertificated learning, which may often involve considerable effort and expertise, is disregarded. In addition, people often have only a limited functional notion of what their actual work tasks involve. Once you come to recognise that learning is infinitely transferable, you will quickly find that you have a vast store of knowledge and skills to bring to your profile.

How long will it take to complete?

In constructing a profile, it is important to have a structure to work within. However, understanding the different ways in which you wish to use your profile will help you to set one or a series of deadlines for completion. Work on the profile at your own pace, based upon your needs and deadlines. Your profile should become a valuable record of learning which you will wish to return to continuously throughout your career. Building your profile should not be seen as entering a race, but rather as a time for you to spend thinking about your current and future professional development needs.

Who owns my profile?

Your profile is unique to you and will contain personal as well as public information. You have complete ownership of it. Some organisations have now bought profiles for their staff to complete. Whilst this is in the main a positive step, it is important that you establish, from the outset, your ownership of the profile. This means that you retain the right to withhold some of its content. In some cases it might be necessary to clarify this with an employer in advance. If it becomes clear that an employer has the right to demand access to the profile provided, the answer is simple: record all of your private information in a separate file – one bought and owned by you. The NMC, for example, makes it clear what part of your profile it may request to see.

How do I know that the learning I am demonstrating is at the appropriate level?

Clearly not all of what you have learnt is necessarily appropriate for inclusion in your profile. We can all identify learning which, whilst useful in one context, is not useful in another. Before you begin, therefore, you need to make sure that you have a fundamental understanding of the criteria against which your profile is being assessed. To enable this, the professional or academic body that is assessing your profile needs to provide you with clear guidelines and criteria as to what is being expected of you. You can only be sure that what you are demonstrating is of the appropriate standard and quality if you have a clear idea what the standard and quality should be. Most organisations should be able to provide you with a set of guidelines and criteria upon request.

How much information should I include?

It is natural for people to want to include *everything* they know about a topic in their profile, but this is not practical, feasible or sound educational practice. In most academic and professional examinations the questions are narrowly focused. So, for example, when sitting an A-level English Literature examination, students are not asked to repeat everything they have learnt about the nineteenth-century novel. Rather, they are required to answer 3–4 narrowly focused but carefully constructed questions. The same approach is adopted in profiling. The points to remember are:

- It is your learning and not your experience which is being assessed.
- The learning you are demonstrating should be sharply focused against the assessment criteria.
- You are aiming to convince your reader that you can meet the assessment criteria – you are not trying to tell everything you know.

The best profiles, therefore, are not always the most bulky. They are the ones that are *concise* and *direct*. What is essential, however, is that the evidence you provide is authentic – it must be your own work and have meaning for you. This means that you must 'speak with your own voice', using your own phrases and a personal approach to the task. This might at first appear daunting, but, in reality, once you have developed your writing skills and can write with confidence you will find that your own style is far more effective.

What should I do if I haven't written for a long time?

Profiling is not simply about past and future learning: it also provides an excellent opportunity to develop skills and knowledge. Profiling requires you to use a range of different writing skills. These might be grouped as **formal** and **informal**. Formal writing includes essays, reports, letters requesting references, completion of goal and action plans, and development of learning contracts. Informal writing includes keeping a diary or journal, writing to a colleague or friend, and summaries of ideas, thoughts and feelings.

As you begin to develop your profile, you may need to develop a range of writing skills that are new to you. There are two ways in which you can improve your formal writing skills. Firstly, you can buy one of the many books on study skills currently available on the market. This should give practical advice and ideas, especially about writing essays and reports. In the bibliography there will also be some suggested reading. Secondly, you might prefer to enrol for a taught course and share what you are learning with others. Most institutes of adult education and further education colleges provide short study skills courses. Many of these are offered in the evening and a fee is charged. Attending a course is useful because it offers the opportunity to experiment with different forms of writing, to look at other people's approach and to get independent constructive criticism.

Writing is all about presenting your thoughts, feelings and ideas in a way that can be read and understood by others. If this is to be effective, you need to learn how to write using your own words and phrases, and your own voice. This is why informal writing is so important. The process of *reflecting through writing* will help in the process of reflecting on practice. Committing your thoughts on paper is in itself reflective and, as you develop your skills of reflection, so you develop your ability to write with meaning and clarity. Playing around with words, feeling comfortable with what and how you write, is integral to owning and taking responsibility for your development and learning:

> She must learn again to speak
> starting with I
> starting with We
> starting as the infant does
> with her own true hunger
> and pleasure
> and rage.
> (Marge Piercy, in Belenky *et al.*, 1986)

Where can I go for help?

Usually, when studying, you are presented with a curriculum. With profiling, *you* are the curriculum and most of the knowledge, skills and qualities required come from yourself. Finding opportunities to discuss your progress with others has many benefits. It enables you to:

- recognise your similarities and differences with others
- articulate your experience
- receive feedback and positive criticism from others
- explore ways of constructing your profile
- develop your presentation skills
- have a regular focus for developing your profile.

There are many people with whom it would be useful to meet in this way. For example, you might wish to share the development of your professional record with a senior colleague. By contrast, if you are exploring a range of aspects of your professional role, you might want to talk with colleagues at a similar level. Some people find it useful to talk with colleagues they work with on a day-to-day basis. Others find it more useful to find a colleague working at some distance, perhaps in a different environment. When you are exploring personal and/or sensitive issues, you need to find people you trust and who will be sympathetic. Most people choose to use family or friends. However, some find it easier to talk with people who are less involved in their lives, but can be trusted to be confidential.

Increasingly, many colleges provide short courses in profiling most commonly referred to as *Making Experiences Count*. Often these courses are attended by people from a wide variety of professional and non-professional backgrounds. Joining a course has the bonus of a group tutor or facilitator, who should encourage you to keep working. Contact your local library for information on courses that are available in your area.

REFERENCES

Belenky, M., Clinchy, B., Goldberger, N. and Taroule, J. (1986) *Women's Ways of Knowing: The Development of Self, Voice and Mind*, New York: Basic Books Inc.

Hull, C. (1993) 'Making Sense of Profiling', in N. Graves (ed.) *Learner Managed Learning: Practice, Theory and Policy*, Leeds: Higher Education for Capability.

Getting Started: Creating Your Personal Profile

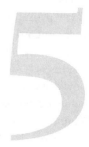

In this chapter you will find practical advice on how to develop a framework for completing your profile. There is information on cross-referencing, layout and presentation. Because writing is an essential part of the process, you will find information on how to develop your writing skills. We also include suggestions on how to write clear statements of competence to support examples of what you can do, together with advice on how to present your work in a way that can be easily understood and assessed by others.

This chapter has been designed to enable you to work at your own pace. You can move backwards and forwards within it, according to which aspect of your profile you are working on. Although we have included activities and practical materials, you will find additional resources in the Annotated Bibliography.

Constructing a coherent profile requires you to be able to carry out a number of different tasks simultaneously. At any one time you may be reflecting upon your past experience, writing letters to potential referees, developing your writing skills, thinking about your future educational needs, and keeping a private record of your thoughts and feelings. Although this might seem daunting, it is actually fairly simple.

This is because each task often dovetails and is dependent upon another. As each section is completed it will be cross-referenced with the rest of the text. Each piece of writing, therefore, needs to be free-standing, whilst at the same time continually integrated with the rest of the material you are producing.

The profile process therefore involves a series of interlocking and yet separate stages which include taking stock, developing a structure, reflecting on past learning, identifying significant learning, proving what you know and can do, and constructing your profile. We will now be exploring each of these in depth. Although activities have been incorporated into the text, additional resources can be found in the Annotated Bibliography. These will give you more ideas for how you can work through each stage.

You do not have to work through each of these stages consecutively. Rather, you should use the sections which best suit your needs as you are working on your profile.

Taking stock

Tell me and I forget
Teach me and I remember
Show me and I understand
(Chinese proverb)

People learn through an active engagement in a four-stage process; this includes personal experience, reflection, making connections between what they are learning and what they know, and experimentation or testing. There are a great many other factors, however, that affect how people learn. These include cultural roots and identity, environmental factors, motivation, previous experiences of learning, emotional and anxiety factors. So, for example, some people may have had bad schooling experiences. They may have been made to feel stupid at not being able to accomplish specific tasks. They may have felt bored and disinterested with school. Their culture and personal identity may have gone unrecognised, and they may have felt confused or isolated by reading texts that had no direct relevance to their own experiences. For some people, then, their experiences of learning have left them with negative feelings about their own capabilities and learning generally. Such people may continue to think that they are stupid, rather than acknowledge the failure of the education system in assisting them to learn. They may believe their early boredom at school signified that they were simply not good at learning, rather than it being the fault of an education system that failed to motivate and challenge.

Beginning a profile allows you to consider how you prefer to learn, to think about what stops you learning and how this can be overcome. You will be simultaneously reflecting upon your experience (of school), working out how you learn best (when the learning is made relevant and recognises your identity), and beginning to create a framework from which to develop your profile.

Reflecting on experiences

Reflecting on experiences can clearly be an enormous task. In the Annotated Bibliography you will find references to materials that will help you with this process, but it is important to remember that you can create your own ways of doing this.

Looking through old photographs is often a useful starting point. Photographs can be the key to unlocking many memories. They may remind you of friends you have long forgotten and places you once visited. They can also reflect your physical changes, moods and the different roles you have undertaken throughout your life. Alternatively, you may find it useful to create a lifeline which charts different aspects of your life such as chronological dates, places you have visited, people you have known, colours and smells you like and dislike, and happy and sad times. The lifeline activity is described in more depth on page 53. If you prefer making things, you may find that you are better able to picture your experiences through painting or sculpture.

Whichever way you approach it, as you begin to put together the jigsaw puzzle of your life, you will find that you remember events you have long forgotten – events that you particularly enjoyed and had meaning for you. This is useful in assessing your learning, as well as in clarifying your aspirations for the profile. Very often people presume that what they formally achieved at school is what they are naturally good at and interested in. But this is not always the case.

CASE STUDY: Marian

Marian joined the profile course because she wanted to be a nursery nurse. As she did not have the correct qualifications, she wanted to use the profile course as an alternative access route. Before she started she said that she wanted to do this because she had been bringing up three children for the last 12 years and felt that she had a lot of experience that would equip her for becoming an effective nursery nurse.

As she began to take stock of her life, there could be no doubt that she did, in fact, have a wealth of relevant experience for nursery nursing. At the same time, however, she began to reflect upon other experiences and interests that she had either forgotten or had not pursued.

This led her to realise that, having brought up children for the last 12 years, the last thing she really wanted to do was return to work to nurse young children. Rather, what she wanted to do was train to become a florist. This was something she had thought about many years previously, but, having raised her children, she had pushed it out of her mind. In fact, she found that she didn't need to complete her profile in order to become a trainee florist. Nevertheless, she found the process had developed her confidence enormously and went on to complete it.

Since then Marian has been offered a job as a trainee florist and has now qualified.

In this case study, Marian's reasons for developing a profile changed as she began to assess her true interests and aspirations. Although she did not need to do so, Marian chose to complete her profile because it had given her confidence. The framework she created, therefore, was very different from the one she originally envisaged, which was organised around meeting the specific criteria for nursery nursing. Her profile acquired a much more personal approach.

At this early stage in the development of your profile, you need to reflect on experiences that you think are important because you:

- think you have learnt a lot
- are pleased with what you feel you have achieved
- have received recognition
- have put in considerable time and effort
- have found the experience either positive or enjoyable
- have found the experience peculiarly negative, or disturbing in some way.

Some of the aspects of your life you might find useful to explore are:

Work   This means thinking about the paid and unpaid jobs you have done

Voluntary activities   This can include involvement in political activities, work with community groups, charity work, public service or fund-raising.

Educational activities   Most people can identify an in-service training course they have attended. However, you also learn from evening classes you have taken, television programmes you have watched, Open University courses studied but not finished, and lectures and seminars attended.

Travelling   This includes travelling for both work and pleasure.

Hobbies   These include leisure activities such as gardening or going to the theatre, as well as more organised hobbies such as sports or playing a musical instrument.

Relationships   Consider relationships that have had meaning for you.

Other   Other aspects of your life worth exploring might include caring for others, books you have read, and projects you have carried out. The list is endless!

As with Marian (in the case study above) your approach to, and goals for, the profile may change during the course of its development. Through reflecting upon your learning, you will come to realise that you are good at many activities, and that you have been in the business of learning for a long time and have learnt a great deal. You will be able to identify many skills and pieces of knowledge that will enable you to access a range of jobs or educational possibilities.

At some point at this early stage, you need to remind yourself of your real reasons for developing the profile. Here are the most commonly cited reasons:

- To clarify my career and/or educational goals
- To gain access to job opportunities
- To gain access to educational opportunities
- To get credit against college courses.

You might wish to include more than one of these reasons in your personal list for developing your profile.

A focus on personal and professional development

Profiling is an excellent opportunity for you to take stock of your life and career in the context of your future educational- and work-related goals. Some people may already have given a great deal of thought to their future career. The vast majority, however, whilst wishing to develop their career, have not spent time focusing on the direction they would like to take.

It is always worth investing time in carefully reviewing your situation and ensuring that the choices are genuine, realistic and achievable. So, for example, Sarah decided that she wanted to do a profile because:

> I have been bringing up children for five years. I have learnt a lot about children and I think I would make a good pre-school playgroup leader. A profile would offer me a chance to get on a course as I don't have the right qualifications.

After reviewing her life and experience, however, she changed her mind:

> On reflection, I have been bringing up children for five years. I now feel it is my time and would like to do something different. Although I do enjoy working with youngsters, I think what I have been interested in all my life, and have never had the chance to explore, is English literature. Perhaps I might be an English teacher one day. (Hull, 1993)

Because most people spend their lives juggling the demands of work and home, spending time thinking about their own needs is a luxury they feel they can ill afford. But taking time to think about who and what you are is important, for both your personal and professional development. It allows you to think about how fulfilled you are at work and whether you wish to move into different areas. Nowadays it is perfectly possible to develop a second career well into your 40s and 50s. As professions change, it is also possible to move into different jobs within the same profession.

Reflection also enables you to make changes in your personal life. You might find that you are unhappy with the balance between home and work. You might be very happy and fulfilled at work but wish you could find a hobby or social life outside of it. At this stage, therefore, you are looking at how the profile process can lead to greater personal and professional satisfaction.

There are many activities that have been designed to help you take stock of your learning and identify your reasons for completing the profile. The following two activities will help you in reviewing your life to date.

ACTIVITY: the lifeline

This will enable you to identify significant events or interests you may wish to explore in the future. Your lifeline will be personal to you and should be kept within the private record section of your profile. It is an activity that can take as long as you feel is appropriate – try not to rush it.

On a piece of paper, represent your life. Do this in a way that has most meaning for you. You might choose to note down important stages and landmarks in your life. You can draw shapes and use colours that reflect important aspects of your life, including places, objects, people and ideas that have influenced you. Some people like to do intricate, colourful drawings, whilst others prefer to draw simple lines or to write. Some use large sheets of coloured paper, whilst others prefer standard A4 white. The important thing is to ensure that it is your personal lifeline that is represented.

Once this has been completed, spend time looking and thinking carefully about what you have produced. Try and identify what is particularly significant to you. It may be, for example, that you have included a particular event that you had long forgotten, but was clearly significant. You may be surprised by what you have left out or how you have represented your life.

This activity is designed to help you to take stock of your experience. It should act as a valuable trigger to memories and past experience, but it should also enable you to recognise how you have grown and developed to date.

The lifeline is something that many people return to continually as they work through their profile. Some update them and reproduce a different lifeline as they continue to develop and learn more about themselves. It is important that each time you have finished working on your lifeline, you think about it and consider what you have gained from doing it.

When making decisions about your future career, you also need to think about the personal values and interests you must satisfy in order to be fulfilled and happy in what you choose to do. Your values affect how you communicate with others and they will have a strong influence on the personal and professional decisions you make. So, you need to take into account what is really important to you when you are making decisions about your career or lifestyle. Of course, values can, and do, change according to age, social and work situation, and interests. Being aware of these changes will enable you continually to reassess which direction you wish your life to take

---

ACTIVITY: professional values

Below is a list of 17 values which relate to professional practice. Some will be more important to you than others. Rank the values in order of importance for you (1 being most important, 17 being least important). You may find that you change your mind continually as you progress.

_____ *Promotion*   Having the opportunity to excel in your job and to be promoted.

_____ *Money*   Earning a reasonable salary; having the opportunity to earn money through overtime and outside of work if necessary.

_____ *Working conditions*   Your day-to-day working environment.

_____ *Hours*   Working hours to suit your needs and interests (this might include weekends, full-time, part-time, etc.).

_____ *Helping clients*   Enabling others to improve the quality of their lives.

_____ *Relationships*   Working as a team; working well with others; developing friendships with colleagues.

_____ *Recognition*   Having your skills and knowledge recognised and appreciated; being taken seriously and given credit for a job well done.

_____ *Learning*   Enjoying learning new skills and knowledge, both outside and within the context of work.

_____ *Security*   Ensuring you have a job that does not carry the threat of redundancy.

_____ *Time*   Having the time to pursue interests outside of work.

_____ *Stress-free work*   Work that is free of pressure, anxiety and deadlines.

_____ *Diversity*   A job that offers the chance to do different kinds of work, and develop new skills and work in different ways.

_____ *Freedom*   Having the freedom to make decisions; to have maximum control over your day-to-day work.

_____ *Admiration*   Carrying out work that others will admire you for.

_____ *Manager*   Managing and organising the work of others; developing policies and implementing procedures.

_____ *Practitioner*   Practising your profession; working with clients, patients and others.

_____ *Other*   Values that are important to you.

Now spend some time looking through the list. What are the factors that may affect the way you approach any future career changes or your professional development? You may find it useful to consider how much your current job fulfils your values and what changes you would like to make in the future.

In this activity you have been looking at values that relate to work and are tangible. However, most values, attitudes and beliefs are not so easy to define because they are more abstract. To gain a comprehensive picture of yourself, therefore, you need to ask questions that help you to understand far more about yourself as a learner and the values you hold. Developing a personal construct grid is one activity that will help you to focus on how you perceive and make judgements about other people. Through this you will be able to focus in more depth on your personal and professional values, attitudes and beliefs.

Profiling encourages you to take stock of yourself in the broadest possible terms. Through construct grids, for example, you will be able to think critically about values and attitudes that inform and underpin your professional practice. In this way, you will not just simply identify your skills and knowledge, you will also come to understand yourself as a learner. This is an essential part of the profiling process. It is our belief that, in order to become an autonomous reflective practitioner, you need to become an autonomous, reflective learner. This means having the ability to reflect upon what you are learning and to make sense of its relevance for you.

Preparation

During this early (planning) stage, there are several factors that you need to consider before beginning work. These are largely to do with time management and creating a learning environment.

Time management

Once you have begun to develop an action plan for completing your profile, you will need to make decisions as to how much time it will take to complete.

If you are using your profile to gain access to a job or course, you will be restricted by an entry or closing date. Knowing that you have to complete your work within a certain time will help you in beginning to plan what can be achieved on a weekly or monthly basis. If you are not restricted by time, you may choose to impose your own deadlines for completion. Of course, you may prefer to work outside a time framework and in a different way. Whatever approach you take needs to be flexible and, most of all, realistic, if it is to be effective. In planning, it is useful to think about the following:

Working life Whether you are working full- or part-time, you need to recognise the amount of time which your working life consumes. This cannot be calculated by the amount of hours spent at work – some people need time to wind up or wind down as they go to and return from work.

Family commitments It is difficult to assess how much time is taken up with the responsibilities of family life. You can work out how much time you spend on chores such as cooking, shopping or cleaning, but finding time to talk with and enjoy the company of close family and friends is much more difficult. Many people find it difficult to create the right balance. You need to allow yourself time to get this right.

Social life Some people may be completing their profile within an agreed time limit. Others, by contrast, will have no fixed limit. Whatever your circumstances, you will need to decide how much time you can realistically give on a weekly basis. Most people are unrealistic when planning deadlines. Because they wish to complete the work as quickly as possible, for example, they drive themselves too hard. So, when they are not able to keep to the deadlines, they feel frustrated and give up.
Allow yourself time to:

- **work**: paid and unpaid
- **rest**: sleep and relaxation
- **play**: with friends and family
- **study**: to complete your profile.

At face value you may feel there is no time left to study, but in reality there is always more time than you think.

ACTIVITY: time management

Make a list of 15 activities that you have carried out over the past month. In this list include daily tasks such as shopping, cleaning and going to the bank, as well as leisure activities such as talking with friends on the telephone, going for a walk or painting a picture. When you have done this, prioritise your activities. Reflect on how much time you have spent on each. Is there a balance between work, rest and play? Can you cut down on the time spent on any of these activities? Can any of them be eliminated?

One way to keep a continuous eye on the time you take to study is to use a 24-hour clock grid:

12 1 2 3 4 5 6 7 8 9 10 11 12 1 2 3 4 5 6 7 8 9 10 11
Mon
Tues
Wed
Thurs
Fri
Sat
Sun

Use the grid to help you keep a record of how you spend your time. On a weekly basis, work out how much time you have spent studying. Think about when and where that study has taken place. Has it been concentrated in one- or two-hourly bursts, or have you attempted to fit in your study at 15-minute intervals? Are you spending more than two hours studying at any one time? Most of all, continually reflect on the effectiveness of your study time. Try and work out new ways of working that are best suited to you and your personal situation. This may mean juggling your existing patterns of waking and sleeping.

Once you have decided how much time you will spend developing your profile, you then need to decide when to study. Some people prefer to get up early each morning, others prefer to work into the night or at weekends, while many prefer to keep the weekends free to play and relax. Whatever you decide upon, try and stick to at least one fixed point on a weekly basis. This will give you a realistic structure from which to develop.

Environment

Creating your own space to read, write and learn is important. You may be lucky enough to have a study of your own, but, if not, you can create a personal space in your bedroom, dining or spare room. Creating a workspace means thinking about what makes you feel relaxed when you want to learn. This might simply mean putting personal photographs or artifacts on your desk or table. You might prefer a cluttered desk or a table with nothing on it at all. There are no right or wrong answers. What is important is that you feel you are working in your own space, free from interruptions and surrounded by things you need to enable you to study. If it helps, put a *do not disturb* notice on the door during your study period.

Developing a structure

Most people have an idea of the deadline for completing their profile. This might be linked to the date for:

- re-registration
- submitting an application to join a course
- submitting a job application.

Once you know the date for submitting your profile, you will be able to develop a realistic framework for work. You need to work out what needs to be done and how this can be achieved – referred to as the development of a critical pathway. Remember, when doing this, you need to allow time for holiday, social and unforeseen events. Each profiler will have a different way of tackling the task. Your plan might look something like this:

Submission of profile for entry to degree course at Maryfield College: 1 October

20 September
- Submit profile: 1 week early!

15 September
- Final typing
- Revise profile
- Check references, language and accuracy
- Check all testimonials are in

10 September
- Share final draft with partner/colleague or academic friend

Summer holidays

30 August
- Complete profile

2 July
- Plan construction of the profile: sequence of work/what should be included

30 June
- Sharpen up writing skills
- Review progress

Complete goal and action plan to identify strengths and areas of weakness
- Include strengths in profile
- Include reasons why courses applied for will enable weaknesses to be addressed

20 June
- Begin writing required competencies, skills

10 June
- Identification of specific knowledge and skills relating to competencies and knowledge required by college

9 June
- Ensure receipt of all documentation, including list of competencies, or guidelines and regulations from the college
- Feedback from academic friend on writing skills
- Practise writing in reflective journal

20 May
- Submit new piece of writing for critical review by academic friend

18 April
- Begin writing for references and testimonials

10 April
- Complete goal and action plan to identify and work on strengths and weaknesses in relation to competencies required by the college

18 March
- Begin identifying personal knowledge, skills and experience in relation to competencies and knowledge required by college

Easter holidays

3 March
- Begin understanding competencies and knowledge required by college

15 March
- Work on developing writing skills
- Complete one written piece of work to personal satisfaction

28 February
- Complete activities relating to identification of skills, knowledge and experience

5 February
- Assess effectiveness of personal writing
- Identify where you can go for extra help

12 January
- Begin developing confidence in writing skills
- Write three different pieces of work in reflective diary

10 January
- Spend time reflecting and taking stock of your past experiences, knowledge and skills

- Think about what you have learnt from your experience

5 January
- Begin goal and action plan to identify why you are applying for this course
- What do you need to achieve before completing your profile?

If you have not studied for a long time you might feel you need to brush up or develop your writing skills. Your reflective diary should help you to practise different writing styles and to discover how you prefer to write. There are also many study skills books available to help you (see Annotated Bibliography for more information). However, it is important to remember that the profile is about you and your learning – any writing and reflective skills used should be yours and not copied from a book. Writing informally in your Learning Journal should help you to develop your preferred writing style.

Reflecting on past learning

By now you should have identified why you want to complete a profile and which one will be used, planned your time, created your own personal space, and begun to identify what skills you will need to work on. You should now be able to move into the next stage of work, which we have called 'reflecting on past learning'.

Until now you have been taking stock of your past experiences whilst, at the same time, looking to your future personal and professional goals. The benefits of this are enormous and should not be underestimated. For many it is the first time they have been encouraged to think about themselves in this way. As one woman said, 'My secret dream is that one day I shall go to college. I told my husband this once and he laughed. He thinks college is for brainboxes. This is the first time I have begun to think it might become more than a dream' (Hull, 1993).

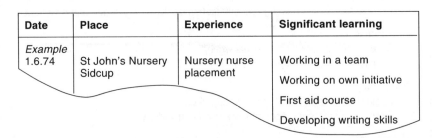

Date	Place	Experience	Significant learning
Example 1.6.74	St John's Nursery Sidcup	Nursery nurse placement	Working in a team Working on own initiative First aid course Developing writing skills

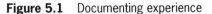

Figure 5.1   Documenting experience

Experience	Key factors	What I learnt	Using what I have learnt
Example Working as a nursery nurse, St John's Nursery	Looking after children Introducing children to new ideas and ways of playing together Working as a team with other workers Time management Management of self	How to work on my own initiative Some basic skills in facilitating learning Much better at working in a team Better at dealing with crises	Bringing up my own children As a student, able to cope with working under pressure In seminars, much better at learning from and with others Organising my time Listening to others

Figure 5.2   The development process

At this stage, you will begin to identify the knowledge and skills you have gained from these experiences. Remember, it is not the experience itself that is important, but the learning you have gained from it. Clearly, much of what you have learnt from your experiences has been acquired unconsciously or unintentionally. So, until you spend time carefully thinking and reflecting upon a specific experience, you may well be unaware of how much you have learnt.

You may have already begun to identify some experiences that appear to have been significant for you in some way. For example, as we noted earlier, many people find that their childhood experiences of school can lead to either a negative or positive attitude towards future learning opportunities. It is these 'significant experiences' to which you need to turn your attention. It is often useful to 'brainstorm' the experience to find out how it has significance for your profile. Figures 5.1 and 5.2 will provide a useful guide in helping you to achieve this.

Identifying significant learning

You will then move on to discover the nature of the learning that has taken place. In thinking about the experience, you want to identify:

- **knowledge**: what you know
- **skills**: what you can do
- **qualities**: which underpin your knowledge and actions.

At this stage you are doing this primarily in order to assess yourself and to determine your objectives for completing the profile. In the Annotated Bibliography you will find some resources to help you with this process. However, it is not always easy to analyse experiences in this way. Here are three of the most common difficulties expressed.

1   How do I recognise that learning has taken place?

Much of what you learn occurs unconsciously, unintentionally and outside of formal education and training. So, even when you think about it, it is not always clear what you have learnt from an experience. Until you begin to reflect critically upon your experiences you will remain unaware of the extent of your learning. As we have said repeatedly, reflection is therefore a crucial element in the learning process and the more you practise the better you become at it. By far the most effective way of reflecting is through journal and diary writing. We discuss this in more detail in Chapter 6.

2   How can I determine the level of my learning?

Clearly, the depth and breadth of your learning will vary depending upon the nature of the experience and the extent to which you have been able to conceptualise and reflect. Learning is largely referred to in levels when it is applied to education and training programmes. The onus is upon the particular awarding body or organisation to clarify the criteria for each level or standard and the skills, knowledge and qualities that are included. When you have a clear idea of this, you can then begin to identify which level your learning can be matched up against. We discuss levels of learning in more depth on page 66.

3   I do not know how to articulate my learning

One of the most common remarks made by those constructing a portfolio is 'I know what I know but I simply cannot write it.' You may have had a similar experience when trying to draw a picture or play a musical instrument: your hands will not do what your brain is telling them. In reality, this usually means you need to understand more about the nature of the activity and to develop your skills. The key in representational drawing, for example, lies in looking at what is in front of you. Without this skill you will find that when you try to draw a tree, rather than representing what you see, you will create your *idea* of a tree. This is a very different form of art! One of the key skills in constructing a profile is the ability to communicate in different ways and at different levels. Remember, your profile is essentially an act of communication between yourself and another person or persons.

Making connections and testing learning

Through profiling you are being encouraged to reflect upon your experiences from new and different perspectives. This, in turn, can lead you to recognise learning that you may otherwise have overlooked. However, the learning you identify is not always easy to categorise or fit into a logical list of skills and competencies. This is particularly true when the profile process challenges you beyond what you actually did, to think about the learning you needed in order to do it. If, for example, you can say that you have effectively managed a speech therapy clinic at your local health centre, you are also being asked to think about what skills or knowledge you need in order to manage a speech therapy clinic. You might identify some of the following:

- **knowledge**: of speech therapy
- **understanding**: of the needs of your clients
- **ability**: to organise your time in order to meet with each client
- **ability**: to write reports, fill in forms and communicate with other colleagues.

The list is endless – managing a speech therapy clinic is clearly a complicated task. When you are producing your profile, therefore, you need to be clear as to which skills, qualities and knowledge you are seeking to identify. As APEL increasingly becomes part of professional development and national credit systems, more and more organisations should be able to describe clearly the kinds of knowledge, skills and qualities which are required in a profile. The criteria can refer to the outcomes of learning or to the process of learning itself.

As you begin to identify what you have learnt from your experience, you will begin to make connections between this new learning and your existing theories, ideas and knowledge. Learning then becomes more than a narrow, personal view or feeling. Rather, you are connecting it within a much broader framework of knowledge. In academic terms, you are 'conceptualising'. This does not mean that your learning no longer has personal meaning. Indeed, it often assumes greater significance, as it is integrated not only with your existing knowledge but also with your personal values, attitudes and beliefs. As with each stage of the profile process, it can also lead to new learning. Let us look at how this works in practice.

CASE STUDY: John

In recalling his childhood, John, a nurse, wrote about being brought up by his grand-mother. He described his grandmother as 'full of life' – an intelligent, articulate woman who had championed many causes and undertaken numerous voluntary activities. He said that she was 'more than a mother to me' and that from her he had learnt to respect and give love to others. At this stage his memories were happy and positive. However, in later life his grandmother suffered from a form of senile dementia. John said that she 'no longer appeared to be the woman he had known', but he continued to respect and love her, just as she had taught him. At times they still shared 'special moments' of closeness. There were also times when he could sense her real pain and anxiety as her sharp mind was made aware of her situation. At this stage his memories were much sadder and less positive. What John found particularly disturbing was watching how the professional staff caring for her no longer treated his grandmother with respect. When she was there they would talk about her, but not to her. Decisions were made on her behalf with no explanation. They would speak to her in tones that were patronising. John saw a rapid decline in his grandmother's spirits. When she died he said that she had simply 'lost the will to live'.

Reflecting on this experience, John felt angry about the way his grandmother had been treated. As a nurse he began to connect this experience with his knowledge and experience in caring for the elderly. He started to read papers and articles on care in the community. He came to recognise that not all those caring for the elderly have shared his experience and are sensitive to the needs of others. He came to realise that his professional practice had been informed largely by the values, attitudes and beliefs he had acquired through experiencing his grandmother's illness and subsequent death. At this stage John was making connections between his personal experience and a wider framework of knowledge by:

- reflecting upon his experience
- attending to his feelings about that experience
- identifying what he had learnt from the experience
- relating what he had learnt to theories, knowledge and ideas
- talking his ideas and theories through with others, including colleagues and friends
- reading papers and articles to gain a broader perspective on his experience.

As demonstrated in this case study, profiling is very much concerned with the current learning which you acquire:

- through reflecting upon your past experiences
- as you develop the new skills needed in order to construct your profile, such as communication skills and techniques in reflection and self-assessment
- as you develop new theories and ideas from reading beyond your personal experience.

However, your knowledge and skills are not wholly learnt until you have tested them out in some way.

> One must learn by doing the thing
> For though you think you know it
> You have no certainty until you try.
> (Sophocles)

For your learning to 'be truly learnt' it must be borne out in practice. You can do this in a variety of ways. At times people choose to test learning in 'real life' situations. For others this raises ethical issues and they might choose instead to conduct experiments which simulate the conditions. Very often you will choose a combination of both. You have many options including:

- writing an essay or report
- conducting an experiment (work-based or other)

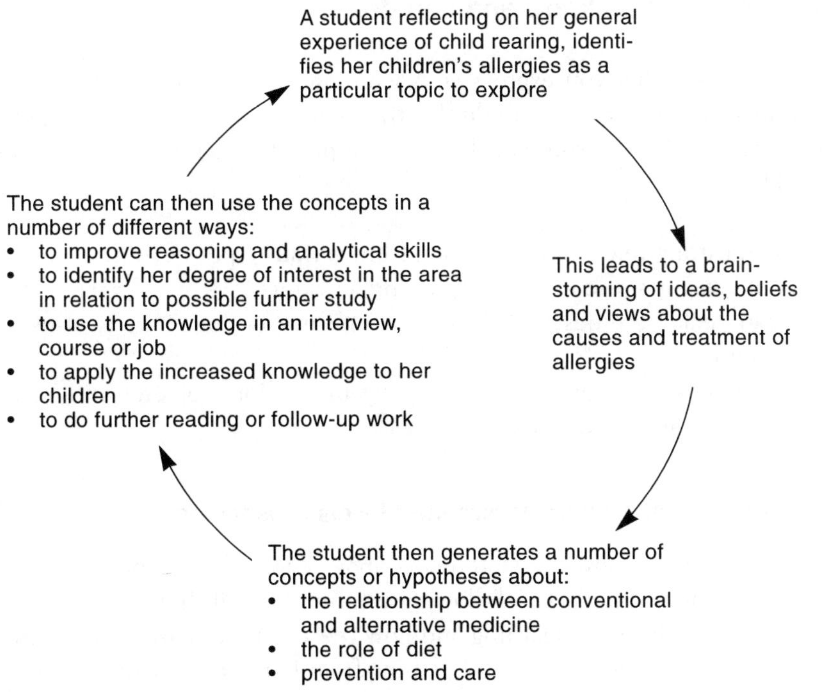

A student reflecting on her general experience of child rearing, identifies her children's allergies as a particular topic to explore

The student can then use the concepts in a number of different ways:
- to improve reasoning and analytical skills
- to identify her degree of interest in the area in relation to possible further study
- to use the knowledge in an interview, course or job
- to apply the increased knowledge to her children
- to do further reading or follow-up work

This leads to a brain-storming of ideas, beliefs and views about the causes and treatment of allergies

The student then generates a number of concepts or hypotheses about:
- the relationship between conventional and alternative medicine
- the role of diet
- prevention and care

Figure 5.3 Example showing how development through the profile process can be related to the learning cycle

- drawing a picture
- role playing.

The option you select will depend upon:

- your preferred methods of learning
- the nature of the learning you are reinforcing
- ethical issues
- whether you are learning independently or have a group of peers with whom you can act out your ideas and theories
- the criteria against which your learning is to be assessed.

In the Further and Higher Education (FHE) Curriculum Development Project, Judith Hinman and Maggie Hollingsworth use the example shown in Figure 5.3 to demonstrate how development through the profile process can be related to the learning cycle we have just been discussing (FEU, 1987).

Proving what you know and can do

It is important that you express your learning in a way that indicates your learning competence. You can do this by writing clear statements supported by examples of what you can do. An example of a statement of this kind could be:

1   I can extract relevant information from various types of sources, such as books, reports, the media, graphs and accounts;
2   I can decide the best way to present information for a variety of uses or purposes;
3   I can present information effectively in the form of oral and written reports, graphs and statistical tables.

Producing competence statements: levels of learning

You might wonder how the statements above can reflect a specific level of learning being claimed. The following information will help you to understand different levels of learning and how these can be written into competence statements (adapted from Learning from Experience Trust, 1988).

1   Knowledge of facts
This relates to knowledge of such things as:

- specific facts (e.g. dates, events, places, etc.)
- definitions
- classifications
- criteria
- methods of organising data
- principles
- theories.

What you know
You may be able to say, 'I know:

- the countries in the EC
- the principles of management
- the definition of a contract
- how to solve problems.'

What you can do
What can you do with this knowledge? At the most basic level, you are able to tell others what you know, so you are able to say, 'I can:

- list/name/specify/enumerate the countries in the EC
- recount/repeat the principles of management
- define a contract
- state the techniques of problem solving.'

---

2   Interpretation of factual knowledge
This is rather higher level of learning, because now you can interpret the facts you know both for your own benefit and that of others. It addresses the question, 'Do I understand?'

What you understand
You may answer, 'I understand:

- the EC
- the principles of management
- the definition of a contract
- how to solve problems.'

What you can do
So you are able to say, 'I can:

- describe the countries of the EC
- restate/explain the principles of management
- explain the definition of a contract
- explain the techniques of problem solving.'

3   Application of knowledge
You may be able to go further and apply what you know to concrete situations.

What you understand
'I understand:

- the EC
- the principles of management
- the definition of a contract
- how to solve a problem.'

What you can do
'I can:

- draw a map of the countries of the EC
- locate the EC countries on a map of the world
- apply the principles of management to my department
- draw up a contract
- give examples of a contract
- solve different types of problems.'

4   Analysis of knowledge
At a higher level, you may be able to analyse the knowledge you have (i.e. break it up into its constituent elements) in a variety of ways and for a variety of purposes. Consider the question, 'Can I analyse what I know?'

What you know and can do
You may answer, 'I know how to analyse what I know in that I can:

- compare and contrast the countries of the EC
- distinguish, appraise and debate the principles of management
- analyse, examine and criticise the definition of a contract
- compare different techniques of solving particular types of problems.'

5   Synthesis of knowledge
A still higher level of knowledge may be reflected in the ability to bring together different elements of what you know and present them in a new way, or create a different framework for them to produce a new idea. Consider the question, 'Can I put together elements of knowledge for various fields/sources and arrange them so as to produce a pattern that was not there before?'

What you know and can do
You may answer, 'I can produce new ideas in that I can:

- formulate policies
- propose policies for the future development of the EC
- teach/redesign the principles of management
- develop new ideas about management
- redefine a contract
- suggest modifications to a contract
- develop new ways of solving problems.'

6   Applications of knowledge

Here you are in a position to evaluate or judge material by applying criteria of various kinds to it. Consider the following questions. 'Can I assess the value of what I know?' 'Can I make judgements about what I know?'

What you know and can do

You may answer, 'I can assess what I know in various ways. For example, I can:

- assess the EC in the light of political, social and economic theories
- evaluate/appraise the principles of management
- assess the validity of a contract
- judge the effectiveness of a contract in protecting against business risks
- decide the effectiveness of different approaches to problem solving, both in theory and in practice.'

ACTIVITY: levels of learning

Below are listed six common learning skills:

- organisation of time
- setting personal objectives
- communicating with others through written reports, memorandums, etc.
- communicating with others orally
- problem solving
- information management.

Select one of these that you feel you would like to present in your profile. Using the information on levels of learning above, try and work out the level to which your learning most corresponds.

To help you initially, you may wish to practise writing a simple statement against each level under the following headings. Consider what you know and what you can do at each level.

1   I know: . . . .
. . . .

2   I can interpret knowledge: . . . .
. . . .

3   I can apply my knowledge: . . . .
. . . .

4   I can analyse my knowledge: . . . .
. . . .

5   I can synthesise my knowledge: . . . .
. . . .

It is important to remember that this exercise simply provides you with a benchmark. Each organisation will have guidelines and regulations to help you.

Constructing your profile

Once you have begun to gather evidence of your learning and experience and documented it in a way that can be understood by others, you will be ready to put your profile together. Some institutions will have their own requirements as to how your profile should be presented. However, in the main, the structure and organisation of your work will be left up to you. When making decisions about what to include and how to organise your work, you should bear in mind the following:

Be selective   Only include material that is relevant and directly connected with the assessment criteria against which your learning is being measured.

Be clear and concise   Make your profile easy to read and understand. Organise your profile logically and allow the reader to move easily from section to section. Use consistent terminology; for example, do not refer to a 'critical incident' in one place and then 'critical analysis' in another.

Be coherent   Make sure that each section connects logically and easily with the next. Make connections between each section if necessary – do not introduce new material in a way that will encourage the reader to ask 'Why on earth has s/he included this?'

Consider the presentation   Your profile should be well presented. If at all possible, type your work and make sure it is accurate, clearly written and grammatically correct, using the same style and format throughout.

Contents

Although your profile will be unique, it will nevertheless contain elements that are common to all profiles. You may wish to bear these in mind when you are drawing up your draft plan.

Introduction   This should provide a brief introduction about you, your reasons for submitting your profile and how these relate to your current or future career or educational aspirations.

Details of your professional experience, knowledge and skills   You will probably wish to outline your career to date, with details of your past jobs and experience, including any unpaid work and voluntary work. Within this you can document your formal qualifications, as well as any courses you have attended that have not been formally credited. There is also scope to include information on articles you have written, research projects you have undertaken and other work-related experience. You can refer back to this information at any time throughout your profile.

Private record   There are some parts of your profile that you will wish to remain confidential. These may include pieces of writing, poems and drawings. You can use this part of your profile to take stock of your past learning, identify your weaknesses, reflect on what you are learning and test out new knowledge.

Competencies, skills and knowledge in respect of award sought (if using the profile for accreditation)   This will form the main body of your profile. It needs to include an outline of each of the skills, knowledge and competencies against which you are seeking to be assessed, and a detailed description of what you have learnt, together with evidence to support the learning you have described.

Within most courses, students are expected to produce papers, complete essays, give presentations and write reports. So, too, through your profile you are being asked to demonstrate that you really do possess the knowledge and skills you claim. However, your profile offers you the opportunity to do so in a creative way that is unique to you. Should you wish to do so, you can include:

- photographs
- articles, poems or short stories you have written
- computer packages you have designed

- care plans you have prepared
- drawings or designs you have undertaken
- reports you have written
- research you have undertaken.

The list is endless. You will also wish to include letters, testimonials and evidence of any public recognition you have received from others. (This may take the form of an article written by someone praising your skill, courage or bravery.)

As you progress, your draft plan will probably change several times in either its organisation or the topics you decide to cover. Continually review your progress and make changes to any draft plan you have made. This will ensure that you achieve a coherent and consistent profile at the end.

Organisation

Your profile has been written to be read and assessed by others. It is more than likely that the person assessing your work does not know you, or has no clear idea as to your academic ability. It is important, therefore, that your profile is easily accessible, clear to read and easy to follow. In your desire to 'tell everything you know', you may forget that someone has to read and make sense of what has been written. The first tip in organising your profile, therefore, is to include features which will help the reader.

Contents page
This should give the reader the main headings in the text, a breakdown of what will be included within each of these, together with clearly marked page numbering.

Cross-reference section
You will probably find that you wish to refer to the same experience to identify a range of competencies or skills. You may also wish to show the same competence or skill at different levels or for different purposes, throughout your profile. Unless you include a competence or skills cross-reference section in your profile, therefore, the reader will find the material confusing. Include this cross-reference section at the beginning of your profile, highlighting areas you have written about or identified throughout your work that you wish the reader to recognise. Your cross-reference page might look like this:

Identification of competencies in being able to work
effectively in a multidisciplinary team:

- Communication skills – pages 10, 15, 34 and 13
  - Presentation skills – pages 17, 14 and 13

Introduction

The reader will want to know that your profile is authentic – that it is really your own work. The best way of achieving this is by presenting your profile from a personal as well as professional viewpoint. Introducing the reader to yourself and your aspirations is therefore an essential part of this process. The introduction need not be more than a few sheets of A4. Simply tell the reader why you wish to develop your profile, what your future educational goals and aspirations are, and how you think the assessment of your profile will assist you in achieving your goals. You may wish to include photographs or pictures which illustrate your writing. Remember to state clearly your aims for completing your profile.

Identification of learning

This is the main body of your profile and will be used to demonstrate your relevant skills, knowledge and experience. Within this section you will need to include evidence that you can genuinely do what you claim. The person assessing your profile will be particularly concerned with what you provide as direct evidence of what you know and can do. This should take up the body of the text. However, you will probably wish to have your claims ratified in some way. In this section you can include your references and testimonials.

Other information

Some of the following can be incorporated within the body of the profile or in separate sections:

Appendices   These might include testimonials, references and a bibliography of publications.

Samples of work   This refers to work that cannot be incorporated within the main body of the text but which enhances what you have written, such as a newspaper article you have written, details of a workshop for which you have been responsible, or details of a campaign you have organised.

Samples from your reflective diary   You might also wish to show the extent of your personal and professional development through the process of producing your profile. This would be very useful if you were submitting your profile for professional development purposes. You may include topics you have written about, observations made, reflections upon the profile process, and development of specific skills (e.g. writing).

Sample framework

By now, you should have decided on the structure of your profile and are beginning to work on different aspects of it. The draft for the contents of your profile, therefore, might look like this:

1   **Introduction**
    Introduction about me
    Who I am
    Why I am producing a profile
    My experience, goals and education/professional aspirations/needs

2   **An introduction to my skills, knowledge and abilities**
    My professional record
        Past jobs
        Past experience
        Qualifications
        Articles written
    My private record
        Personal knowledge acquired through professional practice (i.e. committees, organisational membership outside of work, articles written)

3   **Competencies, skills and knowledge in respect of award sought**
    Communication skills
    Skills in critical reflection
    Ability to work on own initiative

4   **Indirect evidence**
    Testimonials

5   **Appendices**

As you progress your draft contents will probably change in either organisation or topics covered.

Writing skills

Most people, when they begin their profile, are concerned that they have not written in this way for a long time and are not good at it. Bear in mind that you are not being asked to write in exam conditions. With practice, profiling will enable you to write creatively and effectively in ways that genuinely reflect what you know, feel and can do. The best place to practise writing is in your reflective diary. This is because it is a private place and will allow you to try out new ways of writing, make mistakes, experiment with new words and ideas, and discover new ways of organising and presenting your work. We explore this in more detail in the next chapter.

REFERENCES

Further Education Unit (1987) *Assessing Experiential Learning*, London: FEU.

Hull, C. (1993) 'Making Sense of Profiling', in N. Graves (ed.) *Learner Managed Learning: Practice, Theory and Policy*, Leeds: Higher Education for Capability.

Learning from Experience Trust (1988) *Levels of Learning: A Learner's Introduction to Building on Your Experience*, London: Learning from Experience Trust.

Profiles and Reflective Practice

6

> The reflective practice movement has been influential in the way profiles are being used within the profession. This chapter explores some of the theories that underpin reflection. It also offers some practical structures that can be used for reflective practice, which will be particularly useful for those who are just beginning.

It would be difficult to write a book about profiles and not include a chapter on reflective practice. Some would argue that the whole purpose of a profile is to develop reflective skills. Whether you agree with this view or not, it is impossible to ignore that being able to reflect on what you do as a professional is becoming increasingly important, and that you are expected to record those reflections in some way – often within a profile or portfolio.

It will not be possible to cover all there is to know about reflective practice in this chapter. Books that explore the subject of reflective practice in greater depth and breadth are listed in the Annotated Bibliography. We aim to give you a working knowledge of what reflective practice is, how it could contribute to improving your practice, how to approach reflective practice as a skill and how to use your profile to record your reflections.

Reflection and reflective practice are terms that have become increasingly popular and important for many professions, including nursing and midwifery, since the early 1990s. Reflection is becoming recognised by nurses and midwives as an essential component of professional practice, particularly since the popularisation of Schon's book, *The Reflective Practitioner*. Schon (1983) was not the first person to write about reflective practice, nor has he written particularly about health care professionals. However, his work, along with that of Boud *et al.* (1985), Dewey (1933) and others, has been influential in the way nursing and midwifery have embraced the subject of reflective practice.

Reflective practice has moved from a passing fancy or 'bandwagon' (as it was described by critics in the early 1990s) to a central theme that runs through most nursing curricula. It is part of the NMC's standards for post-registration education and practice (PREP), and is central to the nursing policy on clinical supervision. All of this suggests that the reflective practice movement is growing in strength and influence, and can no longer be ignored.

Role of reflection in professional practice

Why is reflective practice important to professional groups and considered to be a part of professional development? Schon (1983) explored the nature of professional practice and tried to explain the role reflection can play in professional action. He recognised that professional work is exceedingly complex and often fast moving, with decisions needing to be made about the best alternatives as you go along.

He suggested that different professions shared common characteristics:

- Professionals face complex problems in their day-to-day work. There are often no definitively right or wrong answers, but only good and not so good ones.
- When making decisions, professionals draw on a knowledge base that is broad, deep and multi-faceted.
- The context in which professionals use their knowledge and skills is very important.
- Professional knowledge is not just about having expert skills.
- It is often difficult for professionals to say or write about what they know and how they use their knowledge.

Clarke, James and Kelly (1994) argue that Schon's real contribution to professionals was to reveal how they cope with these complex problems and what part reflection can play in that.

Schon talks about two types of reflection: reflection-on-action and reflection-in-action. Reflection-on-action occurs when practitioners actively look back and think about an aspect of their practice, and by doing so gain a greater understanding of themselves and the actions and decisions that they took. Reflection-in-action occurs during practice, when practitioners use their learning from previous similar experiences and apply it to their current situation. They are drawing on knowledge they have gained from previous experiences and have internalised, although they may not be able to articulate it at the time. This is sometimes referred to as tacit knowledge. The learning from similar practice situations is used to make sense of what is happening now.

Reflection and learning

As you will have realised from what we have said so far, reflection can lead to learning taking place. If you learn something from reflection, it then gives you an opportunity to use that learning to change your practice or behaviour in some way. The learning can lead to relatively simple changes. For example, you may realise that one way of carrying out a nursing skill is more successful than another; as soon as you have realised that, you can choose to do it in the new way from then on. The learning that occurs can, however, be more complex and personal. For example, you may realise that certain types of patient always seem to annoy you because they remind you of comoone in your paot.

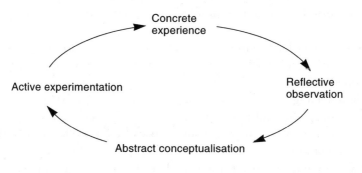

Figure 6.1   Kolb's learning cycle

The connection between reflection and learning is often explained by the use of Kolb's learning cycle (see Figure 6.1). You may have already come across this if you have studied the subject of learning from experience (experiential learning). The basic steps are found in other similar models, such as Gibbs' reflective cycle (see Figure 6.2).

These models identify the various stages people pass through when learning from experience and are useful learning tools in themselves. However, they often represent a false picture – in the real world, the stages identified in the cycle do not operate as such a smooth process. The diagrams imply that one stage always leads to another, but in reality all experiences are not transformed into general concepts, all concepts are not analysed, and not all concepts are tested out in the world. Sheckley and Keeton (1994) realised that the cycle is subjected to the influence of the person who is trying to learn from his or her experience. They believe that

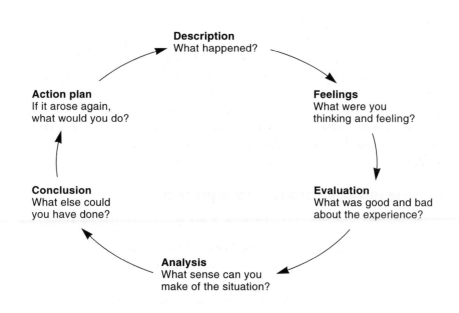

Figure 6.2   Gibbs' reflective cycle

people act as 'information processors' who quickly grasp ideas that confirm
personal views and beliefs, but resist and possibly reject ideas that do not
confirm existing viewpoints. To illustrate their theory, Sheckley and Keeton
have adapted Kolb's learning cycle, as shown in Figure 6.3.

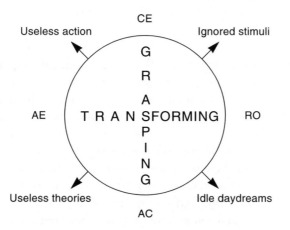

Figure 6.3   Sheckley and Keeton's learning cycle

Remember, any model is just a way of representing something – in this case how you can learn from experience. These models provide a theoretical explanation of why it is that you can learn from experience and the part reflection can play in that. If you find them useful, then use them to help others understand. If you find them unhelpful, then there is no need to worry – you do not need fully to understand or accept them to be able to reflect. They may make sense when you feel more comfortable with your reflective skills, and it may be worth looking at the models again at that point.

Defining reflection and reflective practice

There have been many attempts to define reflective practice. Some definitions are more helpful than others. Have a look at the following popularly quoted ones and decide which makes most sense to you.

> Reflective practice can be interpreted as being the practitioner's ability to access, make sense of and learn through work experience to achieve more desirable, effective and satisfying work. (Johns, 1995)

> The process of internally examining and exploring an issue of concern, triggered by an experience, which creates and clarifies meaning in terms of self, and which results in a changed conceptual perspective.
> (Boyd and Fales, 1983)

> Systematic enquiry into one's own practice to improve practice and deepen one's understanding of it. (Lucas, 1991)

These definitions tell you that reflection is about thinking, learning from your experience and making use of that learning in the future. If you are to become a reflective practitioner, you have to use that learning to expand your professional knowledge to the benefit of your patients, and yourself.

Whilst reflection and some of the theories that lie behind it are relatively new, thinking about what you have done in your professional practice is not. When nurses and midwives first start to read about reflection and reflective practice, they often say, 'but we are already doing this; what's new about this?' Of course, in talking about reflective practice no one is suggesting that nurses and midwives have not thought about their practice before. Schon, by describing how professionals behave, was not inventing a new way of behaving; he was uncovering and exposing behaviours that had gone on before, and trying to make sense of them by giving them a structure and framework. He wrote about this so that others could benefit from what he had found.

Reflection is a process that allows you to uncover and expose actions, thoughts, feelings and behaviours that are present during a period of time. You can use this process to look at any aspect of your life where you want to understand more about what you do and how you can develop. Through understanding more about your professional practice – why you use certain interventions and in what situations – you can extend your personal professional knowledge beyond that found in text books or published research. It is this potential to extend professional knowledge that makes the process of reflection much more than just thinking about practice.

Reflection and profiles

Most of the commercially available profiles address the issue of reflection and reflective practice. At its simplest, a profile provides a storage place for some of the written outcomes of reflection. But many profiles do much more than that by encouraging and explaining the skills of reflection. For example, the Emap Healthcare Open Learning *Profile Pack* encourages you to keep a reflective diary. The authors believe that a continuous process of reflection is an effective way of developing personally and professionally because it can help you to:

- understand the complexity of your work
- analyse your experience and view it more critically
- value your experience
- develop a sense of ownership of your professional development
- confront and think through 'upsetting' incidents
- create an agenda for discussion with others
- appreciate your own development by seeing changes over time, which can lead to an increase in confidence.

If you are following a particular study programme, it is becoming increasingly likely that there will be requirements for you to maintain a profile and (or within it) a reflective diary. Sections of this diary may form part of the assessment scheme for the programme and this should be made clear to you at the outset. The diary's contribution to the assessment scheme may be about demonstrating your reflective skills, or it may be about demonstrating how you are using the outcomes of your reflections in practice.

The implementation of PREP requires nurses, midwives and health visitors to maintain a Personal Professional Profile throughout their career. For this, the development of reflective practice skills will be helpful. The PREP Handbook (NMC, 2002) explains how you can record your learning and reflection, and gives sample case studies using both formal and informal learning. It also involves a template that can help you to think about how to record it.

Profiling is a continuous process that breaks down into three steps:

- Step 1 is about reviewing your experience to date.
- Step 2 is about self-appraisal.
- Step 3 is about setting goals and action planning.

Self-appraisal (step 2) relies heavily on the concept of reflection-on-action, and *The PREP Handbook* gives a brief framework of questions that you can use to reflect on a particular aspect of your practice. When thinking about the NMC requirements for profiling and reflection, it will be important to refer to this handbook. It gives you information about the minimum amount of this type of activity you will need to record in order to success-fully re-register.

The NMC randomly audits a sample of registrants each year to ensure its requirements are being met. Self-appraisal of professional performance is one of the areas where it may request information about your:

- strengths and weaknesses
- achievements
- analysis of significant events through reflection-on-action
- development needs.

Writing and reflecting

The process of reflection does not have to be written down. It is possible to reflect inside your head, rather like doing mental arithmetic. However, our experience has shown that more insights are gained if writing is involved.

The action of writing is useful for several reasons:

- It means that you get the thoughts out of your head and onto paper, where they can be examined and analysed in a less personal and more objective way.
- The process of constructing words and sentences gives structure to your thoughts and recollections.
- A written account gives you a permanent record, which you can read immediately or at a later date to gain further insights.

- If you write on a regular basis and record significant events at the time they happen, this will provide an accurate record to work with.

The whole point of reflective practice (which includes writing things down) is so that you can learn from your professional practice. Walker (1985) has devised, through the experience of working with students, some useful tips on gaining the most from your reflective writing:

- Be frank and honest in your entries. Write it as it is, not as you would like it to be. Be open and sincere in what you record.
- Have a positive approach to the profile. Recognise the potential that it has, and approach it as something that can give you things in return.
- Be spontaneous. Do not spend a lot of time working out what you are going to write, just get something down on paper. It is very useful simply to write and then reflect on what is written.
- Feel free to express yourself in your profile in ways other than writing. Use diagrams, pictures, drawings and other types of material. Sometimes a picture can express what you are trying to say more effectively.
- The profile is meant to be a workbook. Use underlining, circling or highlighter pens to draw out things of significance. As your profile builds up, it is important to go back to the early entries and to reflect further on them.
- Be spontaneous – use your own words to express what you are thinking, feeling and realising. You are not writing an essay that will be marked or making an entry for the Booker prize, so do not worry about the way that you write.
- Be prepared to change your style of working with the profile. Feel free to try different methods – discover your own style.
- Take up the issues that surface when you are working with the profile. Do not get distracted by other more trivial things.
- Persevere in the face of initial difficulties; be faithful to it.

Confidentiality

As we are encouraging you to write down information about yourself and your patients and colleagues, it is important that we address the issue of confidentiality. There are two aspects to consider when considering confidentiality: how to protect your patients and colleagues, and how to protect yourself.

As Walker suggests, it is important that your writings are honest and spontaneous. Whilst writing reflectively, you should not have to be concerned about who might read it. If you are, you may start to censor what you are writing to avoid offending the people concerned, or make any feelings you express suitable for public consumption. If you take this approach, because you are concerned people will read your profile, it is likely to reduce what you gain personally from the writing process.

It is important to remember that no one has the right to read your profile without your permission. The NMC reminds registrants that 'your profile contains confidential information about you and should, therefore, not be accessible to others without your permission'.

When deciding whether to give your permission, you need to understand their reason for wanting to read it. Knowing the reason behind the request will enable you to select parts of your profile that are relevant to their interest.

For example, in *The PREP Handbook* the NMC specifies which parts of your profile it may request to see at the point of you re-registering. It is making it clear in advance of a possible request, so that you can organise your profile accordingly and screen out any aspects that are not of interest to the NMC or areas that you would not wish to disclose. You might consider dividing your profile into two parts: one that contains strictly confidential information; the other that contains information which the NMC may require for audit purposes.

It is now quite common for students completing pre- and post-registration programmes to be asked to keep reflective diaries as part of the programme, sometimes as part of the assessment scheme. These reflective diaries can be part of a profile or asked for as a stand-alone item. The programme organisers should make this clear at the outset and you should be clear what is going to happen to any parts of the diary that have to be given in during the programme. Will it be assessed? If so, what are the criteria for assessment? How many people will see your diary entries? How will they be stored? Will they be copied? Will the copies and the original be returned to you in the future?

When writing about patients and colleagues, it is best not to identify them by name. Documenting any information which could in any way identify patients, clients or carers this could constitute a breach of confidentiality.

It is also important that writings within a reflective diary are not taken out of context, particularly if you are really trying to be open and honest in your reflections. For example, you may have written about a colleague who had made you really angry, and the expression of your anger has been full and free in your diary entry. Having expressed the anger and worked it through, you learn something new about yourself and realise that the colleague was not the one responsible for your anger. Anyone reading your diary entry who did not understand the whole context of the situation, including what you had learnt from it, may well be left with the impression that you do not get on with that colleague. An understanding of the context of reflective writings is essential, and you should consider this when deciding what to disclose to whom.

Reflection – how do you do it?

Learning to reflect and learning from those reflections is a very individual process. There are many useful structures available – examples by Johns (1995) and Holm and Stephenson (1994) are outlined below – but, according to L'Aiguille (1994), reflection can only be learnt by having a go. Some people are more naturally reflective than others, but reflection is a skill that can be learnt, practised and refined by anyone.

In the following section we are going to provide guidance on reflection for those who have no or very little experience of the subject. It is much easier, when starting out, to grasp the skills of reflecting on situations from the past – what Schon (1983) called reflection-on-action. The five main steps to the reflective process are:

1 Set aside time to reflect in a place where there will be no distractions
2 Choose a situation or event to reflect upon
3 Critically reflect on the situation or event
4 Identify areas of learning and decide on any necessary follow-up actions
5 Revisit and re-evaluate.

We will now look at each of these in more detail.

Step 1 Set aside time to reflect in a place where there will be no distractions

Find a place which is comfortable and private, with no distractions. You will need writing materials. At first you may find that any piece of paper will do, but if you are going to keep a reflective diary on a regular basis, then buy a book to write in so that everything can be kept together.

It may take some time to work through the steps in the process, so you will need to set aside at least 2–3 hours. You can break off between the steps and return if you want, but this is easier to do once you become more familiar and comfortable with reflection.

If you speak to colleagues who are already using reflective skills, you will probably find they have a special place, book design or pen they use when making entries in their reflective diaries. This may sound strange and unnecessary, and to some extent it is, but making the process special in some way shows how they value it – and, in turn, how they value themselves. Keeping a reflective diary needs a lot of motivation and commitment, and some people find it easier than others. Find out over a period of time and through experimentation what works best for you. If that means writing with a special pen or in a special place, use it!

Step 2   *Choose a situation or event to reflect upon*

Most people start by reflecting on a situation from their area of practice. It does not matter how you choose the situation – trust your instincts. If a situation pops into your head for no apparent reason, then do not reject it, choose to work with it. You may have heard that people are asked to reflect on 'critical incidents' and worry that the situation you have thought of is not *critical* enough. People's interpretation of 'critical' is often influenced by the medical use of the word, meaning seriously ill. The situation you choose to work with does not have to be like this. It can be a routine and outwardly mundane situation that you meet every day and are very familiar with. On the other hand, it might be a situation that sticks in your mind for some other reason. The point we are making here is that the situation you choose to reflect on just has to mean something and be significant to *you*.

Critical incident technique was originated by Flanagan – an aviation psychologist – during the Second World War, when the US Air Force needed to select and train air crews as effectively as possible. He defined an incident as 'any observable activity that is sufficiently complete in itself to permit inferences and predictions about the person performing the act'. Flanagan was using critical incidents to observe others, whereas you are using his ideas to observe yourself.

So, having chosen a critical incident or situation to reflect on, what do you do next? You need to recall the details of the situation in your mind's eye and then write about it. Some people find it easier to close their eyes to recall the situation and to replay the scene in their mind, rather like rerunning a video of the event. It is important that you recall as many details as possible, such as:

- Where the event took place
- Who was involved
- What actually happened
- How you were involved
- What your feelings were at the time
- What contribution you made to the situation

- What the consequences of that were
- What happened after the situation.

All of this detail needs to be written down, in whatever way makes sense to you. Remember, the writing is for you to work with, not for someone to mark. You can write in any style and in any way that you find comfortable. The important thing is to try and include as much detail as possible. You are likely to find that writing about one aspect of the event triggers memories of other aspects that you have forgotten. It may also trigger connections with other memories; these connections are important, however disconnected they may seem on the surface, so write them down too.

Some people find they want to draw diagrams or pictures to illustrate the situation they are reflecting on. Do not feel restrained by our initial advice to write about the situation – if you want to draw, then feel free to.

Recalling the situation in the way we have described allows you to stand back and 'observe' the event as it happened. The distance encourages you to be objective.

In recalling the situation you might record the feelings that were present at the time. You might just write about them – 'I felt really pleased with myself' or 'I felt really annoyed' – or, as you are writing about the feelings, you may actually re-experience them. There may be a mixture of positive and negative feelings. The feelings you experience need to be acknowledged by you, so they do not become a barrier to you progressing with the reflective process.

Step 3   *Critically reflect on the situation or event*

Just recreating a situation from your nursing past, however, is not enough on its own. Once you have recalled it, you need to do something with it. Remember that the whole purpose of reflection is to learn something from it and extend your personal practice knowledge base.

Structures for reflection

How can you critically reflect on your actions from the past? It is useful to use some type of structure for this. You may want to create your own structure, but being a beginner it may be useful to use one of the structures that already exist within the literature. Many of the frameworks in the literature are composed of a series of questions to ask yourself once you have recalled the situation you are going to reflect upon. These structures have been devised by people who have had a great deal of experience with reflection and it seems foolish not to benefit from that experience, certainly in the first instance. As you become more confident, you can adjust, adapt and refine their structures to make them more personal and relevant to you.

We are including two structures for critical reflection here. References for others are included in the Annotated Bibliography.

Holm and Stephenson (1994)
This first structure was developed by Debi Holm and Sarah Stephenson, two students who were immersed in reflection over a four-year period. They suggest that once you have recalled a situation, you should ask yourself the following questions.

- What was my role in this situation?
- Did I feel comfortable or uncomfortable? Why?
- What actions did I take?
- How did I and others act?
- Was it appropriate?
- How could I have improved the situation for myself, the patient, my mentor?
- What can I change in the future?
- Do I feel as if I have learnt anything new about myself?
- Did I expect anything different to happen? What and why?
- Has it changed my way of thinking in any way?
- What knowledge from theory and research can I apply to this situation?
- What broader issues, for example ethical, political or social, arise from this situation?
- What do I think about these broader issues?

Johns (1995)
This second structure was devised by Chris Johns, who has experience as a researcher, teacher and facilitator of the reflective process. He calls it a 'model of structured reflection'. As well as asking questions about feelings, it also considers the background to the experience and factors that influenced the way you acted. Another feature of this model is that it asks you to think about alternative choices you could have made, and the implications of the experience for your own learning.

For the questions about learning, Johns has been influenced by the work of Carper (1978). This suggests there are four distinct areas of knowledge needed by nurses and midwives:

- Empirics
- Aesthetics
- Ethics
- Personal.

Empirics refers to the science of nursing, aesthetics is the art of nursing, ethics is the moral component, and personal refers to the personal relationship that exists between nurse and patient. These are sometimes referred to as Carper's four 'patterns of knowing'.

Model of structured reflection
Core question: What information do I need access to in order to learn through this experience?

Cue questions
1.0   *Description of the experience*
1.1   Phenomenon – Describe the 'here and now' experience
1.2   Causal – What essential factors contributed to this experience?
1.3   Context – What are the significant background factors to this experience?
1.4   Clarifying – What are the key processes (for reflection) in this experience?

2.0   *Reflection*
2.1   What was I trying to achieve?
2.2   Why did I intervene as I did?
2.3   What were the consequences of my actions for:
  • myself
  • the patient/client/family
  • the people I work with?
2.4   How did I feel about this experience when it was happening?
2.5   How did the patient/client feel about it?
2.6   How did I know how the patient/client felt about it?

3.0   *Influencing factors*
3.1   What internal factors influenced my decision making?
3.2   What external factors influenced my decision making?
3.3   What sources of knowledge did/should have influenced my decision making?

4.0   *Could I have dealt better with the situation?*
4.1   What other choices did I have?
4.2   What would be the consequences of these choices?

5.0   *Learning*
5.1   How do I now feel about this experience?
5.2   How have I made sense of this experience in light of past experiences and future practices?
5.3   How has this experience changed my ways of knowing?
  • Empirics (What does it tell me about the science of nursing or social care?)
  • Aesthetics (What does it tell me about the art of nursing or social care?)
  • Ethics (What does it add to my understanding of moral issues?)
  • Personal (What does it add to my understanding of myself and my relationships with patients or clients?)

Johns is constantly refining this structure in the light of his experience with students and practitioners. If you find the whole model too daunting and theoretical at first, then use the parts of it you feel most comfortable with.

Individual or group work

You can choose whether to use a structure on your own, with a trusted friend or friends, or in a reflective practice group facilitated by a suitably experienced person.

Johns (1995) argues strongly for the benefits of reflecting in a group or with the support of a facilitator, rather than on your own. His work and research show that reflecting can be very difficult to do without expert guidance and support. Being in a group should be supportive, and you can often learn as much from the reflections of others as you can from your own. The group is also likely to be facilitated by a skilled person who can help and guide you with the reflective process.

In addition, a group situation brings the opportunity for supportive challenge from other group members, which prevents you being unrealistic in the conclusions you draw from your reflections. In other words, the group gives you the chance to check whether your perceptions of yourself and the way you acted in a situation are the same as their perceptions. Whilst there are no right or wrongs here, alternative viewpoints can provide learning opportunities.

Whilst supporting the view that an expert facilitator can bring a different approach to reflection, not everyone has access to such a facilitator or group. To meet the NMC requirement, all practitioners will have to learn the basic skills of reflection, using the self-appraisal questions outlined in *The PREP Handbook* (NMC, 2002).

Step 4   Identify areas of learning and decide on any necessary follow-up actions

This step is crucial in the reflective process and yet a lot of people fail to 'convert' their reflections into learning. It forms the major difference between genuine reflection and what nurses have always done when thinking about their practice. At this stage, you should actually begin to identify what you have learnt from reflecting on a critical incident, or what you need to learn before participating in this type of care again. It is important to learn from your successes as well as your difficulties. What worked well in a situation? Does that type of approach/intervention always work well? Is it possible to generalise from this situation to others?

Compare what you have learnt from your own practice with information from other professionals and the literature. See if what you have discovered through reflection is borne out by the theories, techniques and research of others. This fits very well with the Lucas (1991) definition of reflection, which talks about 'systematic enquiry into one's own practice to improve that practice and deepen one's understanding of it'.

If your learning from reflection – which makes up your own personal professional knowledge base – is borne out by others, then this can be helpful as it gives your learning a professional (contextual) validity. If the literature does not support what you have found, this does not mean you are wrong. It may give you ideas to investigate the subject further when you have the opportunity. A literature search may reveal insights or solutions to situations that you would like to improve or change.

Step 5   Revisit and re-evaluate

It is helpful to revisit your reflections from time to time. Of course, this comment assumes that you are keeping a record – written or otherwise – of your reflections and any follow-up actions you decide to take. Revisiting these records is helpful for a number of reasons:

- It can help you realise how far you have travelled since you started to reflect (or from the last time you revisited your journal). It is always satisfying to see your own progress.
- It can help you to identify any patterns in the things you have been working with through the reflective process. For example, do the critical incidents always involve communication difficulties, or difficulties with a particular technique? Does this pattern tell you anything about an area of continuing education you may need to follow?

Ideas for further work on reflection

As we said at the beginning, there is much more to reflection than this chapter can cover. The art and science of reflection is being refined all the time as more people work with it, write about it and share their experiences.

There are several things you can choose to reflect on when you become more confident with the skills, such as:

- Major trends in your career, and whether you are satisfied about the way things have gone
- The way you interact with other members of the multi-professional team, and what contribution you make
- How you deal with constructive criticism and feedback from peers

- How you have coped with challenges and dealt with areas of your practice that need improvement
- How you have made the best use of your talents, qualities and strengths.

These examples can be very challenging at first, because they explore personal issues about who you are and how you respond. However, we encourage you to try out some of the ideas once you feel more confident.

REFERENCES

Boud, D., Keogh, R. and Walker, D. (1985) *Reflection: Turning Experience into Learning*, London: Kogan Page.

Boyd, E. M. and Fales, A. W. (1983) 'Reflecting Learning: Key to Learning from Experience', *Journal of Humanistic Psychology*, 23, 2, 99–117.

Carper, B. (1978) 'Fundamental Ways of Knowing in Nursing', *Advances in Nursing Science*, 11, 13–23.

Clarke, B., James, C. R. and Kelly, J. (1994) 'Reflective Practice: Reviewing the Issues and Refocusing the Debate', unpublished paper given at the 1994 Macmillan Open Learning Conference on Clinical Nurse Specialists, Nottingham.

Dewey, J. (1933) *How We Think*, Boston: DC Health & Co.

Flanagan, J. C. (1954) 'The Critical Incident Technique', *Psychological Bulletin*, 5, 327–58.

Gibbs, G. (1988) *Learning By Doing: A Guide to Teaching and Learning Methods*, Oxford: Further Education Unit, Oxford Polytechnic.

Holm, D. and Stephenson, S. (1994) 'A student's perspective' in A. Palmer, S. Burns and C. Bulman *Reflective Practice in Nursing: The Growth of the Professional Practitioner*, Oxford: Blackwell Scientific.

Johns, C. (1995) 'The Value of Reflective Practice for Nursing', *Journal of Clinical Nursing*, 4, 23–40.

Kolb, D. (1984) *Experiential Learning: Experience as a Source of Learning and Development*, New Jersey: Prentice Hall.

L'Aiguille, Y. (1994) 'Pushing back the boundaries of personal experience' in A. Palmer, S. Burns and C. Bulman *Reflective Practice in Nursing – The Growth of the Professional Practitioner*, Oxford: Blackwell Scientific.

Lucas, P. (1991) 'Reflection, New Practices and the need for Flexibility in Supervising Student Teachers', *Journal of Further and Higher Education*, 15, 2, 84–93.

Mezirow, J. (1981) 'A Critical Theory of Adult Learning and Education', in M. Tight (ed.) *Learning and Education*, Kent: Croom Helm.

Nursing and Midwifery Council (2002) *The PREP Handbook*, London: NMC.

Palmer, A., Burns S., and Bulman, C. (eds) *Reflective Practice in Nursing: The Growth of the Professional Practitioner*, Oxford: Blackwell Scientific.

Schon, D. (1983) *The Reflective Practitioner*, New York: Basic Books Inc.

Sheckley, B. and Keeton, M. (1994) 'Learning From Experience' unpublished paper given at 1994 International Experiential Learning Conference, Washington, DC, USA.

Walker, D. (1985) in D. Boud, R. Keogh and D. Walker *Reflection: Turning Experience into Learning*, London: Kogan Page.

Making Your Learning Count

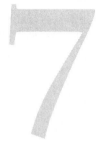

The profile you develop will largely be determined by the academic, professional and/or accreditation framework you are developing it against. In this chapter, therefore, we begin by exploring the concept of accreditation as it is currently used within health and social care education, training and development, and we suggest a working definition. We then move on to look at the implications this has for your own working practices. In this chapter we explore the meanings behind the following terms in depth: National Vocational Qualifications, Assessment of Prior Learning, Assessment of Prior Experiential Learning (APEL) Care Standards.

As we have emphasised throughout this book, there is an increasing awareness within the public and private sector of the need for practitioners continually to develop skills and knowledge that will allow them to maintain professional competence. This, in turn, has meant finding ways of giving formal recognition to what is already known and can be done, regardless of whether this knowledge has been achieved through a formal course of study or informally and through life experience. This is especially true if you work in health and social care where you want to utilise the core skills and experience you have developed since initial registration, whilst also wanting to gain new knowledge and ideas that will improve your practice.

Giving recognition to and valuing informal as well as formal learning is now established within education programmes and accreditation frameworks. Indeed, as educational providers have come to recognise the link between learning and experience (theory and practice), increasing emphasis is being placed upon developing flexible approaches to learning that enable students to develop skills and knowledge relevant to their personal and professional needs. Flexible learning should allow you to have more choice about the content and method of assessment as well as where you learn and the pace at which you choose to study.

All of this is important for several reasons. Firstly, it means that you no longer have to give up work in order to study for a substantial qualification. Secondly, you do not have to re-learn what you already know and can already do, so your learning can become more challenging and relevant. Thirdly, it allows your learning to be recognised wherever and however it has occurred, such as informally through life and work experiences. Finally, it means that you are now better able to plan your learning to fit in with existing work and family commitments.

The emphasis on flexible learning has, in turn, created a need to develop more flexible approaches to the process of accrediting learning. Before we begin to explore some of these flexible frameworks for credit, we need to clarify what we understand by the term accreditation.

Towards a definition of accreditation

A simple definition of accreditation is that it is the process of giving formal recognition or validation to skills, knowledge, experience and competence. In short, it is giving public recognition to what you know and can demonstrate. However, the term accreditation is also used to apply to an organisation or institution's ability to uphold specific standards, and to the process of approving awards. In the broadest sense, then, the term accreditation can be used to describe the assessment and certification arrangements for particular programmes of study and awards, as well as the outcome for you as a learner. Within any definition of accreditation is also the recognition that the process includes interpretation. So, submitting your learning for credit suggests that there is a decision making process regarding what evidence should be caught in assessment and what information recorded in certification:

> Recognition of skills, competence or knowledge is not merely a passive or dispassionate acknowledgement that they have been attained. It implies an evaluative judgement about their worth – crudely, a granting of market value. The process of consideration of this market value often relates to what the trainer, teacher or supervisor decides to record on the final certificate. This act of interpretation by the receiving party is as much a part of the accreditation as the processes which go into creating those statements. (Further Education Funding Council (FEFC) 1999)

It might be useful at this point to remind you that although assessment and accreditation are closely connected, they are not the same. Whilst learning cannot be accredited without being assessed, clearly learning can be assessed without being accredited. Credit is gained through the achievement of learning outcomes and their assessment

Accreditation of continuing professional development

Continuing professional development (CPD) is the term most commonly associated with the ongoing learning that you need to undertake throughout your career in order to maintain your professional knowledge and skills. There are several national accreditation schemes, which recommend the development of a profile in order to accredit the professional knowledge, and skills you have acquired since you began your practice. We look at the principles and practices behind each of these schemes, particularly National Vocational Qualifications, Open College Network's accreditation framework, and the higher education Credit Framework system. However, there are other flexible accreditation systems and we provide website addresses for these on page 107.

National Occupational Standards

National Occupational Standards (NOS) have been in existence for around twenty years. NOS are statements of competence designed to describe performance – what you are expected to do at work. They are important because they have been designed in partnership with employers, workers, professional bodies and others to highlight the quality of service you are expected to provide. In Social Care, for example, the occupational standards for social care are 'owned' and have been developed by TOPSS in partnership with the General Social Care Council, the National Care Standards Commission (whose work includes regulating the staff training requirements of the Care Standards Act 2000), and the Social Care Institute for Excellence which provides research in particular social care settings.

In short, NOS describe best practice.

Individual professionals and organisations are free to use National Occupational Standards as they wish and for a variety of reasons including:

- by you as a professional to enable you to develop your knowledge and skills, and improve the care you provide
- by educational and training organisations so that they can provide courses that are relevant to improving practice
- by accrediting organisations in order to design qualifications
- by employers for designing jobs, recruiting staff and career planning and appraisal.

For further information on National Occupational Standards see www.skillsforhealth.org.uk

In the care sector, the purpose of developing NOS is to improve the quality of service that patients/clients receive, by making clear the quality of care those who provide it are expected to perform.

Clearly, health and social care jobs are not easy to break down as they rarely involve tasks that do not, in some way, relate to each other. Health and Social Care Occupational Standards, therefore have been designed to reflect a holistic view of care that also recognises the values or concepts of patient/client centred care.

National Vocational Qualifications

The historical context

During the 1980s, there was growing concern about the lack of vocationally related education and training offered to people both inside and outside work. It was because of this that a wide range of national schemes and programmes, aimed at improving and extending vocational education and training, was established.

With all this in mind, the National Council for Vocational Qualifications (NCVQ) was established in 1986. Now referred to as NVQ, it is an independent body, funded by the government. It has no legal powers and can only effect change with the cooperation of the awarding bodies, industry bodies, professional bodies and further and higher education.

About NVQs

NVQs are qualifications about work. They are based upon standards of competence set by industry. Because they are competence based, it is meeting the standard that is important. So long as you are able to demonstrate that you have met the standard, you can expect to the get the credit. There are no barriers. Access to NVQ assessment is open to all. There are no discriminatory rules or age limits.

NVQs are based on National Occupational Standards, which, in turn, are statements of performance that describe what a competent practitioner should be able to do in a particular job. The Standard Setting bodies set these National Occupational Standards.

So, NVQs are defined in terms of competence in specified performance. Being competent is not seen as referring to a low or minimum level or performance. Rather, it refers to the standard required *successfully* to perform an activity or function. So, as a competent practitioner you are performing to professional or occupational standards.

Each NVQ is given a title and a level to locate it in the NVQ framework. The NVQ framework is a way of showing how qualifications relate to one another and how you can progress through the system. There are five levels in the framework – level 1 being the most basic – as follows:

Table 7.1 National Vocational Qualifications Framework

Levels	Definitions
Level 1	Competence that involves the application or the performance of a range of varied work and which may be routine and predictable
Level 2	Competence that involves the application of knowledge in a significant range of varied work activities, performed in a variety of contexts. Some of these activities are complex and non-routine and there is some individual responsibility, or autonomy. Collaboration with others, perhaps membership of a work group or team, may often be a requirement
Level 3	Competence that involves the application of knowledge in a broad range of varied work activities performed in a wide variety of contexts, most of which are complex and non-routine. There is considerable responsibility and autonomy and control or guidance of others is often required.
Level 4	Competence that involves the application of knowledge in a broad range of complex, technical or professional work activities performed in a variety of contexts and with a substantial degree of personal responsibility and autonomy. Responsibility for the work of others and the allocation of resources is often present.
Level 5	Competence that involves the application of a set of fundamental principles across a wide variety of contexts. Very substantial personal autonomy and significant responsibility for the work of others and for the allocation of substantial resources features strongly, as do personal accountabilities for analysis, diagnosis, design, planning, execution and evaluation

The NVQ levels can also be described as follows:

Level 1: Foundation skills in occupations
Level 2: Operative or semi-skilled occupations
Level 3 Technician, craft, skilled and supervisory occupations
Level 4: Technical and junior management occupations
Level 5: Chartered, professional or senior management

Source: www.dfes.gov.uk/nvq

For more information on NVQs visit the NVQ website: www.dfes.gov.uk/nvq

Key skills

If you have thought about taking a course recently it is likely that you will have come across the words 'key skills'. Key Skills are the skills that all of us use in our everyday life and work and which are essential to any effective learning we do. Key skills include:

Communication
Information Technology
Numeracy
Learning how to learn
Problem-solving
Team building.

Each of these are skills that can be developed at different levels, and most courses are now expected to include them within the curriculum. There is a number of websites on key skills. For further information you might start with www.dfes.gov.uk/keyskills

Awarding bodies

Open College Network credits

The National Open College Network (NOCN) is one of the largest awarding bodies in the UK. There are 28 Open College Networks (OCNs) across the country which provide accreditation for adult learning. OCNs provide qualifications and programmes in a broad range of subjects and work with educational providers such as adult education centres, further and higher education, as well as trades unions and employers to develop accredited learning programmes that are relevant to adults.

OCN accreditation fits into the National Credit Framework. The levels within the National Credit Framework are as shown in Table 7.2.

Table 7.2   National Credit Framework

Levels up to and excluding higher education are:

Level	Description
Entry	The acquisition of a limited range of basic skills, knowledge and understanding in highly structured and self-referenced contexts which permit the identification of progression from the learner's point of entry to the learning process

continued

Table 7.2 National Credit Framework (*continued*)

Level	Description
One	The acquisition of a foundation of competences, knowledge and under-standing in a limited range of predictable and structured contexts that prepare the learner to progress to further achievements
Two	The acquisition of a broader range of competencies, knowledge and understanding that demonstrate the extension of previous abilities in less predictable and structured contexts and prepare the learner to progress to further achievements
Three	The acquisition of a more complex range of competences, knowledge and understanding in contexts which develop autonomous, analytical and critical abilities that prepare the learner to progress to further independent achievements

OCN equivalences with NVQ

In Table 7.3 we show the approximate equivalences between the OCN Credit framework levels and other qualifications.

Table 7.3 Equivalences between OCN Credit Framework levels and other qualifications

Level			
Three	NVQ3	GNVQ advanced	A level
Two	NVQ2	GNVQ intermediate	GCSE A-C
One	NVQ1	GNVQ Foundation	GCSE D-E

Source: nocn.org.uk

For more information on OCN credit visit the NOCN website: www.nocn.org.uk

National Qualifications Framework

The regulatory criteria of the National Qualifications Framework (NQF) took effect in September 2004. The aims of the NQF are to:

- Promote access, motivation and achievement in education, training and professional development
- Promote lifelong learning
- Provide clear progression routes for students
- Avoid duplication and overlapping of qualifications.

The National Qualifications Framework sorts national qualifications into three categories and six levels (entry level to level 5). The levels are shown in Table 7.4.

Table 7.4 National Qualifications Framework

Level	General	Vocationally related	occupational
5	HIGHER LEVEL QUALIFICATIONS		Level 5 NVQ
4			Level 4 NVQ
3 advanced	A Levels and AVCE		Level 3 NVQ
2 intermediate	GCSE A*–C grades	VOCATIONAL	Level 2 NVQ
1 foundation	GCSE D–G Grades	QUALIFICATIONS	Level 1 NVQ
Entry level	CERTIFICATE OF ACHIEVEMENT		

[AVCE: Advanced Vocational Certificate of Education]

The positioning of qualifications at the same level indicates that they are broadly comparable in terms of general levels of learning. They do not indicate that they have same purpose, content or outcomes. The NQF places qualifications into three categories:

General
Vocationally related
Occupational

These categories relate to: attainment in subject (general), attainment in a vocational area (vocationally related), and attainment of competence at work (occupational). Qualifications may incorporate the characteristics of more than one category.

A National Credit framework places the learner at the centre of their learning. It enables them to earn credit for their learning irrespective of its level, the time it has taken or the place it was learned. In this sense, learners get cumulative recognition of their learning as they progress.

For more information on National Qualifications Framework: www.qca.org.uk

Accreditation and your portfolio

The purpose of developing a portfolio is simply to provide evidence of your learning – which might or might not set against occupational standards – in a form which can be assessed by others. Your portfolio will be unique to you. However, the most successful are those that take into account the framework against which they are seeking accreditation. For example, in assembling your portfolio against an NVQ, it is important that it is clearly mapped against the relevant occupational standards, and shows evidence of knowledge, skills and competence.

Claiming credit for your Prior learning

Seeking credit for your informal learning will require you to demonstrate your knowledge and skills in exactly the same way as you would if you were claiming credit for formal learning. However, you may not know or be clear about the extent of your informal learning, and may need to think about your experiences and identify what you have learned. Claiming credit for formal learning involves two stages: (1) Identification of evidence to support claims; and (2) submission of your profile for formal assessment. In claiming credit for informal learning the process involves two additional stages. In this section we take you through each of the four stages involved in preparing your informal learning for academic or professional credit. These stages are very similar to the process of constructing your profile outlined on page 70.

There are four stages involved in preparing your informal learning to submit for academic or professional credit. These stages are very similar to the process of constructing your profile (see Chapter 5).

- Stage 1: Systematic reflection on experience
- Stage 2: Identification of significant learning
- Stage 3: Identification of evidence to support claims
- Stage 4: Submission of profile for formal assessment.

Let us look at each of these stages a little more closely.

Stage 1: Systematic reflection on experience

As you have already seen, reflection is an important part of the APEL process. There are two ways in which you can reflect upon experiences: you can do it close to the time of the event, or you can reflect some time later. Although you are not always aware, some of your most significant learning experiences might have happened a long time ago, perhaps even in your childhood. The first stage in the APEL process therefore lies in systematically reflecting on experience, in order to identify where significant learning has occurred.

At this stage you are simply being asked to recall your experience. The question you are being asked to address is simply: 'What experiences have I had?' Some people find it useful to 'brainstorm' or talk this through with colleagues and friends. Others find it useful to write an autobiography which includes jobs done, people encountered and places visited. This will depend upon the amount of time you have allotted.

This stage is perhaps the most important one in the process because it will provide you with the substance from which you will be working.

Stage 2: Identification of significant learning

Having mapped out your experience in some form, the next stage is to identify what you have learnt from it. This means focusing on the experiences identified in Stage 1, in order to begin making claims about what you have learnt. Often learning claims are offered as learning statements. You will find more about writing learning claims in Chapter 5. Learning claims normally have two elements to them. Firstly, there is a claim to your knowledge at some level. Secondly, you are making a claim to be able to perform a skill or to do something. The form in which you present your claims will depend very much on what you are seeking your learning to be assessed against.

Stage 3: Identification of evidence to support claims

One of the purposes in producing a profile is to provide evidence that you have acquired the learning you have described. It is accepted that students in a classroom must provide evidence of their learning in the form of essays, oral presentations or written examinations. Similarly, in the profile process you will be expected to demonstrate that you possess the knowledge or skills you are claiming. What counts as evidence will again depend on the nature of what you are seeking your learning to be assessed against. For example, someone making a claim for credit against a music course might substantiate the claim by writing and playing a music score. A claim to knowledge in computing might be accompanied by a computer package. If you are working in the area of mental health, your claim might point to an education programme you have devised. So, evidence may take many forms. Broadly, there are two types of evidence: direct and indirect.

Direct evidence
This refers to evidence you have directly created. It might include performance you have given, reports you have written, the assessment of your

clinical practice or work-based experience. In most cases, direct evidence is the most effective in demonstrating that you really do know and can do what you are claiming. Direct evidence can include a wide range of material, such as:

- a report you have compiled and written (in whole or part)
- an article you have written
- the design of a curriculum
- presentations, speeches, talks or training events you have carried out (this can be managed through an audio or audio-visual tape)
- manuals you have written or designed
- photographs
- drawings, graphs, paintings and sculptures you have made.

This list is not exhaustive and you might think of other things that could be included. However, in all forms of direct evidence you need to show that the work really is yours, or demonstrate the part you played in its development.

Indirect evidence

This refers to evidence from others about your claim to learning. It can take the form of:

- a testimonial from someone with expertise in the field, including a supervisor or manager
- letters written on your behalf by colleagues, including a supervisor or manager; a letter might also come from a professional association or an organisation with whom you have carried out voluntary work
- awards you have received
- magazine, journal or newspaper articles about you
- certificates of attendance at courses and workshops.

Avoid evidence which might suggest bias, such as a letter from a family member or close friend. Also avoid letters or articles about events in which you were involved, but which do not mention you specifically or fail to highlight what you did and the skills you used.

Finally, any evidence you offer should be clearly associated with the particular learning claim. So, for example, if you are approaching a colleague for a reference, s/he will need to be briefed as to the specific learning claim you are seeking to address. Without a link being made between the claim and the evidence, it is difficult to give a realistic assessment of what has been learnt.

Summary of assessment

Your completed profile will include both direct and indirect evidence. Within this you should try to include:

- accounts of relevant experience
- relevant certificates/awards
- supporting documentation
- current assessments
- details of an oral assessment.

Stage 4: Submission of profile for formal assessment

Once you have identified your sources of evidence, you need to prepare your profile for submission. Much of the work will already have been done by this stage; your task now is to assemble it, making it accurate and easy to read. How the profile is submitted will depend largely on the requirements of the validating and accrediting body. We discuss this process and offer practical advice in Chapter 5. Although professionals disagree as to what should be included in a profile and the format it should take, the one thing they all agree upon is the criteria by which it will be finally assessed. These are as follows:

Breadth	The learning is not isolated from wider considerations.
Authenticity	You can do what is claimed.
Quality	The learning is at the appropriate academic level.
Currency	You have kept up to date with recent developments.
Acceptability	The evidence supports the learning claim to which it is linked.
Sufficiency	There is enough evidence to show sufficient proof of confidence.

The most important guiding principle of APEL is that you have ownership over your own profile. This means that it is up to you to make claims to have your knowledge and skills recognised. So, it is your responsibility to make a claim and support the claim with appropriate evidence. Although you might need support in order to achieve this, it is important to recognise that APEL is concerned with your ability to engage in self-assessment and ultimately take charge of your own learning.

In some cases your profile will be assessed by just one other person. Usually, however, the assessment of your profile will involve at least two other people, and in many cases it will be carried out by an APEL committee. Whoever is involved in the assessment, it will be their job to read the entire profile, weigh up the evidence of learning, and make judgements as to its value. Sometimes this process will be similar to a formal written examination and you will not be involved in the process. More normally, however, the assessment will involve an interview. In the vast majority of cases this interview is conducted in an informal, conversational manner. It is not seen as part of the formal evaluative/assessment process. Rather, interviews are carried out in the spirit of giving positive feedback to aid your future development.

APEL is the assessment of certificated and non-certificated learning (including experiential learning).

Terminology

Below we have listed a glossary of terms associated with the accreditation of learning, and where appropriate have included website addresses:

Term	Description
CATS	Credit Accumulation and Transfer – this refers to the process of accumulating credits towards an award, as well as transferring accumulated credits across courses and higher education institutions
Level	A description of the level of skill, knowledge and or competence
TOPSS	A registered charity responsible for developing the National Occupational Standards for Social Care www.topss.org.uk
QCA	Qualifications and Curriculum Authority which is responsible for ensuring the standards in education and training. It works in partnership with others to develop the school curriculum and associated assessments, and to accredit and monitor qualifications in schools, colleges and work www.qca.org.uk
Assessment Centres	These are the organisations approved by the Awarding Body to assess NVQs. They may be educational providers, training organisations or employers
Assessors	Professionals appointed by an approved centre to assess the evidence of learning submitted by a candidate
External verifiers	Professionals appointed by the appropriate awarding body to maintain the quality and standards of approved centres

Sector Skills Development Agency	The network that brings together the organisations working with the government to develop the skills of specific sectors of the workforce www.ssda.org.uk

Other awarding bodies

There is a number of other awarding bodies offering accreditation. You will find detailed information on each of the following websites:

City and Guilds:	City and Guilds.com
BTEC:	btec.org.uk
Edexcel:	edexcel.org.uk

Helping Others to Develop a Profile: The Skills of Facilitation

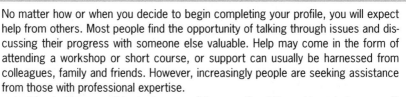

No matter how or when you decide to begin completing your profile, you will expect help from others. Most people find the opportunity of talking through issues and discussing their progress with someone else valuable. Help may come in the form of attending a workshop or short course, or support can usually be harnessed from colleagues, family and friends. However, increasingly people are seeking assistance from those with professional expertise.

In this chapter we will look at some of the specific skills and knowledge you will need in helping someone to complete a profile. We begin by introducing you to some principles about how adults learn and what they bring with them when they embark on a learning programme. We then move on to explore the five key skills of facilitation enabling, educational counselling, advising, assessing, and informing.

If in an educational situation an adult's experience is ignored, not valued, not made use of, it is not just the experience that is being rejected, it is the person. (Knowles, 1984)

This chapter looks at how you can help others to complete their profile. We will explore the specific skills required, as well as some common problems that arise.

In order fully to understand some of these issues, it would be useful for you to understand theories underpinning how adults learn. We begin this chapter, therefore, with an introduction to learning theories that emphasise experience as the source of development. In particular, we look at the importance that the learning process has within the construction of a personal/professional profile, and the relevance of this for professional development.

Learning from experience

The learning that you bring to your working practice has not simply been acquired from formal courses you have attended. Rather, you learn from a broad range of informal learning experiences, such as voluntary activities, leisure pursuits and employment, as well as through family and social situations. So, the learning you use at work is derived from a multiplicity of sources – both at the workplace and outside of work. However, because learning in our culture has so often been associated with formal qualifications, your informal or experiential learning (which often involves considerable effort and expertise) is often disregarded and remains underutilised.

This means that you cannot make assumptions about what you already do or do not know based simply upon your formal qualifications. Rather, you need to find ways of understanding more about yourself as a learner, and valuing and articulating the extent of your knowledge.

Your interest and willingness to learn will be influenced by many factors, including personal characteristics and motivation; the characteristics and requirements of the particular job you are doing; and the nature and culture of the environment in which you work.

Learning cycle

David Kolb is an American writer who has written extensively on this theme. For Kolb, learning is a cycle (see Figure 6.1 on page 78). We have adapted it as follows:

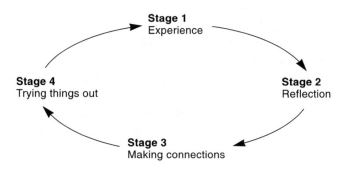

Figure 8.1   Kolb's learning cycle (adapted)

According to this approach, all learning is rooted in experience, but for learning to take place it must actively involve the learner. The emphasis is on learning through discussion, problem-solving and action. What is important in this approach is that the learner comes to internalise what is being learnt in ways that have personal relevance and meaning.

This can be contrasted with traditional approaches to learning, which often promote passive learning gained through the knowledge of an active teacher. This traditional approach is referred to as 'the banking concept' of education; learners are 'filled up with knowledge' which they normally cash in at a later date when they undergo a formal examination process.

Kolb's cycle can be used as a framework to promote learning within the profile process. It brings together theory (reflection/conceptualisation) and practice (experience/testing out), and it can make you aware of your individual approach to learning and learning preference. Understanding *how* you learn is as important as understanding *what* you have learnt, as it helps you to learn more about what motivates or blocks you from learning.

Concrete experience (experience)
In Kolb's learning cycle the learning begins with an experience or event. This might be a specific experience, but it can also include a series of related tasks such as bringing up children or experience of voluntary work. It might also refer to some event you have observed, such as watching a baby being delivered or attending a play or concert.

Reflective observation (reflection)
When you begin to think critically about some of these experiences, you move into the second stage of Kolb's cycle. Although learning is derived from experience, it does not just happen; for learning to take place you need to engage in critical reflection. At this reflective stage, therefore, you begin to identify significant experiences that have the potential to be turned into learning. This involves far more than simply the skills of interpretation. Rather, at its most effective, reflection causes you to ask questions that expand your knowledge and enable you to examine your feelings and values. Through reflection you are able to think carefully about how you approach your work, and thereby extend your professional competence.

One writer who has explored critical reflection in some depth is Jack Mezirow. Mezirow (1983) argues that critical reflection includes the following elements:

- self-examination
- exploring options for new ways of acting
- building competence and self-confidence in new roles
- planning a course of action
- acquiring knowledge and skills necessary for implementing one's plans
- provisional efforts to try new roles and assess feedback
- a reintegration into society on the basis of conditions dictated by the new perspective.

Mezirow calls this process 'perspective transformation'. He argues that perspective transformation provides us:

with the awareness of why we attach the meanings we do to reality, especially to our roles and relationships – meanings often misconstrued out of the uncritically assimilated half-truths of conventional wisdom and power relationships assumed as fixed. (Mezirow, 1983)

Abstract conceptualisation (making connections)

In the third stage, you use reflection to integrate your new experience with previous experience. Whereas in the second stage reflection may have lead you to realise that your experience was an isolated example of a general pattern of behaviour, in the third stage you begin to form ideas or theories about what that pattern might be. In this way your learning becomes shaped by experiences and cultural context, as well as personal values, attitudes and beliefs. This stage is crucial in contributing to individuality and personal identity.

Active experimentation (trying things out)

In the final stage you begin to apply your new ideas to new situations in order to test them out. This stage is particularly important in your professional development, because it provides you with the opportunity to bring together theory and practice. In this way you experiment in ways that may lead to another concrete experience, and so continually move around the learning cycle. You can test new ideas through simulation, role play or in real-life situations. Through role play you can test out theories and ideas without using clients or patients as guinea pigs in the learning process.

Learning style

Experiential approaches to learning recognise that each person has an individual learning style:

As a result of our hereditary equipment, our particular past life experience, and the demands of our present environment, most of us develop learning styles that emphasise some learning abilities over others. Through socialisation experiences, family, school and work, we come to resolve the conflicts between action and reflection between immediate experience and detached analysis in characteristic ways. (Kolb, 1984)

Kolb argues that some people 'excel at assimilating disparate facts into coherent theories, yet these same people may be incapable of, or uninterested in, deducing hypotheses from those theories'. Others may be able to do this, but find it impossible to involve themselves in active experience

Kolb (1984) identifies four commonly occurring learning types:

Convergers These are high scorers on conceptualising ('making connec-tions') and experimentation ('trying things out'). People who exhibit this learning style are said to excel in the application of ideas. They are also characterised as having narrow technical/scientific interests and as being unemotional.

Divergers These are high scorers on concrete experience ('experience') and reflection. People who exhibit this learning style are considered to be imaginative, emotional and interested in people. Their interests are broad and tend to be in the arts.

Assimilators People who fall in this category tend to prefer conceptualisa-tion ('making connections'), together with reflection. They lean toward inductive reasoning, integration of knowledge and the creation of theoret-ical models. Their social interest is not as strong as that of their divergent colleagues.

Accommodators This learning style is typified by concrete experience ('experience') and experimentation ('testing things out'). People who demonstrate this learning style are good at doing things, trying out new experiences and taking risks. Their approach to problems is said to rely on intuition and trial and error, and is likely to involve other people.

One of the major factors influencing people's preferred learning style is, for Kolb, their current job role. This largely refers to the content of the job, but clearly the relationships they have with their colleagues is also an important factor. So, for example, those people who are working in general management jobs that demand a 'strong orientation to task accomplishment and decision making in uncertain circumstances' require an accommoda-tive learning style. Those people who are working in jobs that demand prac-tical and problem solving skills require a convergent learning style.

Increasingly, as the nature of professional practice changes, you will need to acquire different learning styles in order to accommodate the dif-ferent requirements of your work.

Assisting others with their profile

Developing a profile is different from almost any other learning activity, in that the curriculum to be studied is not an outside body of knowledge but the learner her/himself. If you are helping someone to construct a profile, therefore, you may not *start* by pointing to a pile of books and suggesting that s/he reads these to learn more about a specific topic. Rather, at the outset, you will be helping the profiler to make sense of the knowledge and skills s/he has already learnt and can do, and to make decisions about what the profile should include.

In most learning activities there are two elements. The first is the process through which the learning takes place; this is often referred to as the *how* of learning. The second is the content or substance; this is the *what* of learning. In more traditional approaches to education, the content of learning is largely based on external, existing knowledge available to all. In current (experiential) approaches to professional development, however, greater emphasis is being given to the learning which is intrinsic to the learner, and the process through which that learning occurs.

The skills you need to help others with their profile are almost identical to those used in experiential or open approaches to learning. Professionals who use this type of approach may be known as tutor/counsellor, educational guidance worker, mentor, enabler or educational counsellor. In this book we have chosen to use the term *facilitator*. This is for two reasons. Firstly, in our belief it encapsulates each of the different terms identified above. Secondly, it is the most commonly used and understood term in the field of open and experiential learning.

In order to develop your skills as a facilitator, you need to begin by understanding how adults learn and what they bring with them when they embark on a learning programme. Some learners come with preconceptions about themselves and their ability to learn. Some put up barriers which stop them from learning, whilst others open themselves up to new ideas and concepts. So, you need to understand that each learner is unique, with a wide range of experience, knowledge and skills that they will want to identify and explore.

Blocks to learning

The person you are assisting may simply be completing the profile because it is a professional requirement. At worst this might make them hostile to the whole concept; at best they might be prepared only to undertake the bare minimum of work in order to complete the profile.

Some people may feel hesitant about starting because they have not studied for a long time and lack confidence in their knowledge, abilities and experience. Their perception of personal development might be based on their experience of school, where they were perhaps made to feel stupid, or where the information they were learning had little relevance or meaning for them. Certainly, many people who did not perform well at school have been left feeling that education is not for them but for 'clever people'.

Whatever their experience, almost all adults returning to study after a break feel unsure as to their ability to retain knowledge, write for academic purposes, take notes or read effectively. Profiling also raises problems for learners who hold rigid views that have remained unchallenged for a considerable time. Profiling encourages learners continually to question their personal assumptions, values and beliefs about themselves, their profession and the world in which they live.

Challenges to pre-existing knowledge can also present learners with problems. This is particularly true if they are working in a profession where (as in nursing and midwifery) they have traditionally been taught from the received wisdom of others or through direct experience. This is what Rogers (1988) refers to as learning through a 'significant other':

> Any challenge to this learning material, to our existing knowledge implies either a challenge to our significant other (it may be some other respected authority) or a challenge to our self-judgement (we chose to rely on that person, or book, it seemed reasonable at the time) or to both. (Rogers, 1988)

It is also important to remember that most people hold strong beliefs about themselves, their profession and their practice. Through profiling, as people begin to explore and challenge their existing assumptions, they may find a conflict between what they believe about their profession and what they practise; between their personal and professional values and practices. All of this will have implications for how they practise in the future, and it might even lead them to abandon a particular stance or attitude they have upheld in public:

> This will lead some participants to resist learning changes. They will cling to pre-existent knowledge and attitudes and find it hard to assimilate new material or at least not make it harmonize with what is already there. So they adopt mechanisms, most commonly of withdrawal in an attempt to preserve what they already possess. (Rogers, 1988)

Finally, if people are resistant to returning to study, they will identify a host of reasons why their profile will not be successful. Ageing, physical tiredness, declining powers of memory and concentration are all cited as blocks to achievement. Although some may genuinely encounter such problems, research shows that if people are excited, motivated and involved in what they are studying, these factors can usually be overcome. Concentration and memory retention are skills that can be worked on and developed.

Again, however, identifying topics that are personally and professionally motivating will improve both of these skills enormously.

Your first task as facilitator, therefore, is to assist the profiler to remove any blocks to learning and, more often than not, to go through a process of unlearning past experiences of education. If the profiler has many barriers to overcome and does not know where to start, you might need to help by finding exercises which will build immediately upon her/his knowledge and abilities. In this way you will be getting rid of any negative self-image and beginning to instil confidence.

Begin by enabling the profiler to identify what these blocks might be. Through the reflective diary, explore these in a positive way and devise personal strategies for overcoming them. The profiler might wish to talk through ideas with you, show you what s/he has written in the diary, or ask your help in developing an action plan for the future. But remember, it is always up to the profiler to determine what help s/he needs from you in order to develop.

Facilitation skills

Facilitating a profile requires a number of complex and interrelated skills. Below we have identified five key skills which we believe all professionals engaged in profile facilitation should possess.

Enabling

At its simplest, enabling means *supporting* the profiler through the development of her/his profile. It involves a number of skills, the most important of which is *listening*. Most learners need someone who will listen carefully and encourage them to articulate their thoughts and ideas. This is called active listening. It means listening carefully to what is being said, whilst at the same time continually challenging the learner to review, analyse and make sense of what s/he is articulating and thinking. Active listening is not easy. Often you will be tempted to interrupt and give the other person your views and ideas on what is being said:

> For some of us, the greatest difficulty of all is to control ourselves, to listen without intervening. Knowing when to shut up has all sorts of aspects: it means knowing that it may be best to keep silent even though there is a pause. It means resisting the temptation to short-circuit the whole process by giving too many lubricating lecturettes, clever, perhaps,

and even illuminating, but still not as useful as the students finding their own way in their own time. It means, most of all, shutting up so as to listen better until we hear what is really being said behind often clumsily-chosen words. (Rogers, 1986)

Active listening requires that you stop thinking about yourself and your opinions. Rather, it means genuinely listening to what the profiler is telling you.

Another key enabling skill is to create an environment in which the profiler feels able to speak openly and in confidence about what s/he is thinking and feeling. The profiler should never be encouraged to discuss topics which s/he considers to be private or does not wish to share. The skill lies in enabling the profiler to speak freely about issues which s/he is keen to discuss. So, for example, try to arrange the room in a way that will make the profiler feel relaxed and comfortable, and will create a supportive climate for discussion.

Educational counselling

This refers to helping the profiler to discover, clarify, assess and understand her/his learning in order to plan realistic current and future educational aims and career goals. There are many opportunities for adults to get independent career and personal development advice nowadays. And you might want to suggest that where people might find out about services that are available to them. You might begin by looking for information, advice and guidance on the lifelong learning website (www.lifelonglearning.co.uk)

Advising

This means helping the profiler to interpret information and to make decisions based on her/his planned learning needs. It might also involve simple advice on where to go for specific information or how to construct a request for a reference letter.

Assessing

Self-assessment is an essential component of profiling. Through careful facilitation you will be enabling the learner to develop confidence in self-assessment and to evaluate the depth and range of her/his learning. Through self-assessment the learner will be much more likely to take control of the profile, to make informed choices about what it should include and to have ownership of it.

Informing

At times it might be appropriate for you to provide information about learning opportunities and professional development policies that may inform the development of the profile. This should be done in a manner that enables the profiler to make her/his own decisions about the specific merits or options from this information.

Most people find the prospect of taking responsibility and ownership of their profile daunting. Initially, they argue that they would rather be told what to do. In the early stages, therefore, you may find that the learner is expecting you to tell her/him what to do and how to organise the work. Most people also come to learning with expectations about their tutor. Students often come to learning expecting the facilitator to be both an expert and an authority figure. And, indeed, tutors often feel it is their role to impart knowledge and to tell the students what they should be learning and how this might be achieved. They want to solve all their students' problems and provide answers to all their queries:

> The worst forms of teaching are often the nicest because they encourage attitudes towards the students and their abilities which, though well-intentioned, are forms of patronage. Inevitably, there are many variants. The most obvious is the man who is over fond of his own voice, who too obviously likes to hear himself speak. A smile appears on his face as he talks, as though he is actually testing the sound of his own rolling periods; you can recognise the element in yourself by the feeling of almost physical pleasure when you are led into that kind of rhetoric. It's like finding you can fly, for a few yards. Those of us who were brought up in the Nonconformist chapel tradition are especially at risk here – the combination of rhetoric, earnestness and the urge towards charismatic relationships is heady. (Richard Hoggart in Jennifer Rogers, *Adults Learning*, 1986)

This approach, then, creates a climate where the student, albeit unintentionally, becomes dependent on the facilitator to make all of the decisions about what and how s/he should be learning. It does little to enable the learner to understand the extent and breadth of her/his learning and to take responsibility for it, all of which is necessary if s/he is to become a more autonomous, thinking professional through a process of self-assessment and profiling:

> Life at its best, is a flowing, changing process in which nothing is fixed. Life is richest and most rewarding when it is this flowing process. To

experience this is both fascinating and a little frightening. I am at my best when I can let the flow of my experience carry me, in a direction which appears to be forward, toward goals of which I am but dimly aware. In this stream of my experiencing, and in trying to understand its ever-changing complexity, it should be evident there are no fixed points. There can be no closed system of beliefs, no unchanging set of principles which I hold. Life is guided by a changing understanding of and interpretation of my experience . . . There is no philosophy or belief or set of principle which I could encourage or persuade others to have or hold. I can only try to give others the permission and freedom to develop their own inward freedom and thus their own meaningful interpretation of their own experience. (Rogers, 1971)

This initial stage of helping the profiler to move from being *dependent* on the facilitator, to becoming an *independent* learner, is one of the most valuable aspects of profiling. It is through this process that the profiler should come to understand and appreciate the significance of her/his life experience to date and to develop confidence and self-awareness in her/himself as an individual as well as a professional. In short, if the facilitator listens to and takes seriously what the learner wishes to share, then the learner, in turn, will begin to acknowledge the relevance of her/his ideas and knowledge.

Planning the profile

Developing a profile requires very careful planning and preparation. Briefly summarised, there are two planning stages to profiling. In the initial stage, the profiler will be making decisions about whether to develop a profile 'from scratch' or whether to buy one off the shelf. This means s/he will need to think carefully about her/his personal and professional circumstances, and to make decisions about how the materials will be presented and the approach to be adopted. In the second stage, the profiler will make decisions about how the profile should be structured, what it should contain, how long it will take to complete and the range and depth of knowledge to be included.

Planning therefore involves identifying the skills, knowledge and attitudes required by both profiler and facilitator, and establishing the learning goals and the individual tasks that need to be completed in order to achieve these objectives. It also involves identifying what resources will be available. These can be human resources, including use of a facilitator, family and friends, or they can be physical resources, such as use of a library, study area and computer.

You might suggest that the learner spends 2–3 weeks researching what is available by visiting a library, making contact with colleagues and others, and gaining their support.

It is important that during the planning stage the facilitator does not take control. Rather, you should be continually encouraging the learner to take control, identify her/his learning, and make any decisions. This is not as easy as it might sound. Very often as a facilitator it is possible to see all kinds of ways in which your profiler can progress. For example, time and again the profiler will disregard a particular experience as worthless, whereas you might view it as a valuable source of learning. Whilst you might suggest that the profiler 'revisits' the experience to find learning potential, it is always up to the profiler to make connections between learning and experience and decide what s/he wishes to disclose.

It is often the planning stage that is the most difficult. As a facilitator, you need to allow the profiler to take as much time as s/he feels is necessary. However, your task is also to ensure the profile is working within the deadline for completion, and that the profiler has not become 'stuck' and unchallenged. Very often, people beginning a profile find it is the first time they have thought about their experiences in such a structured and positive way. They find it exciting when long forgotten memories are remembered and they are able to see their life as a learning continuum. If this happens, the learner will fiercely resist any attempt to turn newly acquired learning into a set of competence statements, or translate it into a language that can be immediately assessed. One way to ensure that an effective balance is achieved is through negotiating a learning contract from the outset.

Developing a learning contract

Alan Rogers (1988) argues that in most learning situations a bargain is struck between tutor and student. 'The terms of the bargain may not have been spelled out in full, but the agreement is there none the less.' A learning contract is where the facilitator and the learner work out the details of 'the bargain' in full, and negotiate the terms and conditions. For the profiler, this means asking her/himself a number of fundamental questions:

- Why am I developing a profile?
- Do I understand enough about the profiling process?
- When do I need/wish it to be completed?
- What type of profile do I want?
- What skills have I already got in order to complete it?
- What skills do I need to develop?

- How do I want to use my facilitator?
- What help can I expect from others?

The facilitator needs to ask her/himself:

- How much time am I realistically able to give?
- What skills have I already got in order to facilitate the process?
- What skills do I need to develop?
- Does the profiler's view of the ways in which I am able to help, tally with my own?
- What will my role be in this process?
- Where can I point the profiler to get additional support?

Setting goals and criteria for success

It is important that you and your profiler openly discuss these questions first, together with any other issues. This should help both of you to clarify the long- and short-term learning goals. So, for example, one long-term goal will be to complete the profile; one short-term goal for achieving this might be to develop written skills to a personally and professionally satisfactory standard. The profiler may have more than one long-term goal for the completion of the profile. S/he will usually have several short-term goals.

It is very important that the long- and short-term goals are written down and understood by both of you. Alongside these, the best learning contracts include the criteria for success. Successful criteria for the completion of the profile might include the following:

- I have used it to support an application for a job.
- I have used it to gain academic credit against a course.
- It was constructed, cross-referenced and written to a high personal and professional standard.
- I now understand far more about myself and my professional development needs.

Successful criteria for the completion of written skills might include the following:

- I now have confidence in my writing ability.
- I can construct a sentence using my own words and phrases.
- I now understand the writing process.
- My profile is written clearly, concisely and using my own style.

Drawing up an action plan

The second part of writing a learning contract involves the profiler in working out the actions s/he will take, and the timescale for each, in order to achieve all of her/his goals. The action plan for developing a personal writing style might include the following statements:

1   Try different writing styles in my reflective diary. See which style I prefer and why.
    Timescale: Ongoing throughout the profile process
2   Look at a number of different writing styles used by professionals, including newspapers, journals, reports, novels, etc. Analyse similarities and differences between each; see what I like and dislike.
    Timescale: One month
3   Try approaching the writing of my profile in different ways.
    Timescale: Two months
4   Read an article on writing from one of my study skills books.
    Timescale: begin after I have completed actions 2 and 3. Two weeks only
5   Ask family, friends, facilitator to comment on what I have written.
    Timescale: Begin as soon as possible, after two months of commencing my profile
    (Please note: the times are merely an indicator. The timescale will be different for each person depending on their confidence in writing and the timescale for its completion.)

Clarifying the facilitator's role

As the facilitator you will then be in a good position to negotiate *your* terms and conditions. You should discuss the type of support you are able to offer, the amount of time you can give, and the nature of your relationship. An effective profiler–facilitator relationship is one which is an equal partnership. The effectiveness of this equal relationship will affect the quality of the learning experience for the profiler and the outcome of the profile. Your job is primarily to enable the profiler to make the most of the human and physical resources available.

Many profilers may want a more directive relationship, and require you to comment on any written work they have submitted by awarding marks and correcting grammar. It is important when you embark on work, therefore, to explain how you perceive your role and to discuss the need for the profiler to take responsibility for her/his own learning. You may want to indicate that, whilst you are more than happy to comment on work submitted, it is not appropriate for you to correct grammar or award marks in this way. You must carefully explain that, as the facilitator, your role is one of guidance, educational counselling and progress chasing to make sure the profile is completed within the time delineated. But ultimately, it is the profiler who must take ownership of the profile and make decisions as to its development.

This does not mean that you are not able to give your opinion, or to make suggestions as to how the profile can be improved. Rather, it ensures that you are not seen as an expert and authority figure upon whom the learner can remain dependent.

The facilitator and profiler need to organise the context within which the learning takes place. It means thinking about the environment and the conditions in which both you and the profiler can work effectively. Creating the right learning environment will have an enormous impact on the profiler's motivation, attention and achievement.

Remember that this may be the first time the profiler has been encouraged to talk about such personal issues. However well the profiler knows you, s/he will probably feel nervous or apprehensive about doing so. Clearly, then, it is important to create an atmosphere which feels 'safe' and inviting.

In addition, the profiler will not always want to meet with you alone. Sometimes, s/he will wish to meet with peers, colleagues, friends and others to share issues and brainstorm ideas. Will you be able to find suitable accommodation for small group work? If not, can your profiler suggest an appropriate place in which to meet?

David Boud *et al.* (1985) suggest that learners need *freedom to learn*. They need to be free from the pressures of their everyday lives in order to think and reflect. This means that people need to allow themselves space and time to study, but many feel guilty about taking time out to learn. Try and encourage your profiler not to feel guilty. Build sufficient time into your meetings for her/him to block out all the external factors s/he will bring into the room. Find ways of enabling her/him to throw out the 'daily baggage' for a short time.

Establishing ground rules

Creating the appropriate conditions in which to learn also means that both of you need to establish the ground rules within which you can both work. Within a conventionally taught course, the ground rules are much more clear. Each college has a mission statement and prospectus that makes clear to the student what resources are available and what are not. This will include use of computer and library facilities, as well as attendance at lectures and seminars, and tutor allocation and role.

The learning contract is an excellent place for you both to establish ground rules. The profiler will be able to state what s/he wants to achieve and how s/he wishes to achieve it. This in turn means that the profiler is acknowledging responsibility for her/his own learning.

As facilitator, you must make your role equally clear. This means establishing when you are available and, equally, when you are not. You should also acknowledge that in this role you are not a counsellor. This is important. Sometimes, when the profiler is discussing personal aspects of her/his life, this might throw up a specific, emotionally charged experience which s/he has not thought about or confronted before. In this situation the profiler may well need to find someone to talk it through and help her/him to understand or come to terms with it. These kinds of skills are not skills for the facilitator. Rather, you need to point the profiler in the direction of someone who is professionally trained to help.

In addition, you need to clarify any expectations you may have from your profiler. So, for example, you may wish to establish rules about ensuring you both keep to agreed starting and ending times of meetings. Working within an agreed time framework will help to ensure the discussion is more focused and achieves the objectives your profiler has set.

Progress chasing

Perhaps the most important element of facilitation lies in challenging the profiler to move through the different stages of development to completion. This is not as easy as it sounds. Most people find that, once they have overcome their initial fears, thinking about their experience is fascinating and of great interest. They enjoy the process of reflection and of exploring their personal and professional lives. They find it difficult to move into *analysing* what they have learnt from their experience and *documenting* this in a way that makes sense and can be assessed by others.

The learning contract, again, will form a sound framework from which you and the profiler can review progress. There may be legitimate reasons why the profiler is not progressing as quickly as anticipated. The learning contract should be continually renegotiated and new deadlines set. However, your job is to enable the profiler to be honest as to the reasons for any delay, and to identify where there are blocks to progress and how these might be overcome.

Evaluation

Whether you are facilitating or learning, you need to find ways of working out how effective you have been. Evaluation is simply a process of enabling you to do so. Evaluation should enable you to think about your facilitation skills, identify your weaknesses and map out ways of building upon your strengths. Evaluation is an essential component of the learning process.

There are two forms of evaluation, formative and summative. Formative evaluation is the continuous evaluation that goes on throughout the learning process. Summative evaluation is that which takes place when the profile has been finally completed. In reality, of course, both feed into each other. The learner should be actively involved in both forms of evaluation. This is just as true when you are evaluating your facilitation skills. The profiler should be continually giving feedback as to whether you are effectively supporting her/his learning needs.

At the heart of this process are the questions that both facilitator and profiler must address:

- To what extent is the profiler developing and engaging in the profiling process?
- What is the quality and level of her/his development?
- How much of what is incorporated into the profile is owned and understood by the profiler?
- How motivated is the profiler to develop?

Questions for you to ask, therefore, are more to do with how well the learner is developing than how well you are performing as a facilitator.

In this chapter we have highlighted some of the key issues you need to address in facilitating the profiling process. If you would like to explore the subject in more depth there are many books currently available. You will find some suggested reading in the Annotated Bibliography.

===== **REFERENCES** =====

Boud, D., Keogh, R. and Walker, R. (1985) *Reflection: Turning Experience into Learning*, London: Kogan Page.

Knowles, M. (1984) *Andragogy-in-action*, San Francisco: Jossey Bass.

Kolb, D. (1984) *Experiential Learning: Experience as the Source of Learning and Development*, New Jersey: Prentice Hall.

Mezirow, J. (1983) 'A Critical Theory of Adult Learning and Education', in M. Tight (ed.) *Adult Learning and Education*, Kent: Croom Helm.

Rogers, A. (1988) *Teaching Adults*, Milton Keynes: OU Press.

Rogers, C. (1971) *On Becoming a Person: A Therapist's View of Psychotherapy*, London: Redwood Press.

Rogers, J. (1986) *Adults Learning* (2nd edn), Milton Keynes: OU Press.

Further Resources: Further Activities to Help You Develop Your Profile

9

In Chapter 5 Getting Started: Creating Your Personal Profile, we included some activities to help you to begin developing your profile. In this section we include other activities that people engaged in profiling recommend. These are:

- Conducting a personal SWOT analysis: This will help you to identify your strengths and weaknesses, and begin to plan career and educational goals
- Mind mapping: This will help you to identify the skills and knowledge you already have but have perhaps forgotten about, and/or think of opportunities you would like to access
- Developing a goal and action plan: This will help you to write realistic goals and action plans so that you can achieve your educational and/career plans
- Understanding your learning style: This will help you to find out how you learn best – and therefore the type of course or learning activity you might prefer. It will also help you to understand your abilities and strengths as both a learner and at work
- PEST analysis: This looks at the external factors such as political, economical, sociological and technological that you need to think about when planning your future career and educational goals.

ACTIVITY 1: conducting a personal SWOT analysis

SWOT stands for *Strengths, Weaknesses, Opportunities* and *Threats* and it is a simple activity to help you to think honestly about what you are good at and what you need to improve, as well as potential personal and career related opportunities and what will stop you taking them. Carrying out a SWOT analysis, therefore, will help you to assess your skills and plan your future.

Below is a sample of a personal SWOT analysis. However, it's a good idea to do your own before reading this through in depth. On page 127 we explain the steps involved in completing your SWOT.

STRENGTHS
- Motivator
- Creative – able to think outside of 'the box'
- Able to work on own initiative
- Work well in teams
- Supportive of others

WEAKNESSES
- Starter – not a finisher
- Not methodical

- Act first – think afterwards
- Haven't learnt the 'no' word
- Can be seen as too soft

OPPORTUNITIES
- Care of older people more recognised – could work almost anywhere in the UK and plenty of opportunities for promotion
- Sarah and Tom have now left home. More time to devote to career
- chance to study for a degree – which I have always wanted to do

THREATS
- John still working so cannot move too far away.

- Feel more tired these days.

- Need to earn money

- Mum not too well – want to be around to care for her if necessary

---

Having brainstormed your SWOT analysis you now need to study it – and identify what it tells you about a) you and your skills and those you need to update and b) how you might begin developing a goal and action plan for achieving any personal and/or professional goals you might have identified.

There are many ways of interpreting your SWOT analysis. So, in the above example this person might come to the following conclusions:

I would ideally like to go to university. I've always wanted to do it and its 'my time' now. I wonder if I would be able to cope with doing a degree? I haven't written an essay since I was 14. Also, I don't know what I want to study. I love reading novels – but wonder if a degree in English literature will help me get a job. And I want to make sure I have enough time to look after my mother as she gets frail.

I shouldn't forget, either, that I enjoy working in a nursing home and there is plenty of scope for me to develop my practice and earn more money.

Conclusions and action plan

I think I should find out more about what a degree involves and perhaps aim to apply to university in 5 years' time. This will give me chance to continue developing my practice and see exactly what career opportunities might be available to me in the future (I might end up doing a degree in Caring For Older People!). And I can continue to care for my mother now and in the future. In the meantime, perhaps I should find out about short courses that I might be interested in doing. An access course might be a good idea. When my friend Iris did one she really developed her confidence and she learned how to write an essay.

Doing your own SWOT

Use the sheet of paper on page 129 to carry out your own SWOT analysis. Before doing so, however, its worth remembering that most of us are much better at identifying our weaknesses than we are at recognising what we are good at.

Identifying your strengths

Ask yourself:

- What do I do well?
- How would other people describe my strengths?

When identifying your strengths, think about different aspects of your life including:

- Your qualifications – which might include a professional registration, but also identify all the short courses you have attended whether they are accredited or not.
- Your professional experience – which might include a range of jobs both within and external to your work in care. How have your jobs shaped you? What skills have you developed?
- Personal (life experience) – this can include bringing up children, caring for a relative, voluntary work and/or hobbies that have given you new skills, knowledge and ideas.

Imagine how another person might describe your strengths.

Identifying your weaknesses

When identifying your weaknesses do not beat yourself up. A weakness doesn't necessarily mean we are bad at something, or that we are incompetent. It simply recognises that we cannot be good at everything – and some of our skills can be improved or developed. Ask yourself:

- What could be improved?
- What do I do badly?
- What should I avoid?

Imagine how another person might describe your weaknesses.

Opportunities

With the pressures of everyday life it is easy to forget there are more opportunities available to you than you might imagine. When thinking about what opportunities there are try to be as open as possible – don't close an opportunity down before you have had a chance to explore it. Ask yourself:

- Where are the opportunities available to me?
- What are the interesting trends within health and social care which might lead me into a new job?

Opportunities come about for a range of reasons including:

- Advances in technology
- Advances in health and social care
- Changes in government policy
- Changes in society (e.g. demography).

Threats

What factors will stop you achieving what you want? These factors might be practical (e.g. need to earn money/care for family), personal inhibition (e.g. lack of confidence in ability), or other general factors (e.g. do not hold a relevant qualification). Remember: knowing what you want is one thing. The next is working out a strategy for overcoming the barriers to achieving your goal. Ask yourself.

- What are the obstacles to achieving my goal?
- What are the threats to my current job?
- Do any of my weaknesses threaten my current or future work?
- What changes in health and social care threaten me and my work?

Analysing your SWOT

This activity should help you to focus on your strengths and begin to identify how best to tackle your weaknesses. It is also intended to help you to recognise the opportunities available to you and to give you the confidence to achieve your goal.

Once you have completed your SWOT take time to think about the points you have made in each of the areas described. Can you see any connections?

My Personal SWOT

STRENGTHS

WEAKNESSES

OPPORTUNITIES

THREATS

ACTIVITY 2: mind mapping

Tony Buzan introduced mind mapping into the UK over thirty years ago. It is a straightforward activity that offers a creative approach to note taking and problem solving. When finished, your mind map looks like a spider diagram, but it will also contains a lot of thought and a variety of ideas. Put simply, mind mapping is a visual way of capturing a complex topic on a piece of paper. It will help you to see the relationships and connections between key concepts and ideas, and to link relevant information.

Most people write notes in a linear style on a piece of lined paper – using the same coloured ink. When you draw a mind map you use a blank piece of paper (any size and shape) and different, brightly coloured inks. Doing this, according to Buzan, your notes become more attractive to your brain, which in turn will make it work more effectively to capture your thoughts and ideas.
To draw a mind map:

1   Take a piece of blank paper and turn it on its side (landscape).
2   In the middle write the name of the topic you want to mind map. Try to use different colours to make your words stand out. You might not want to use words – you can draw a picture to capture your topic instead.

My important life experiences

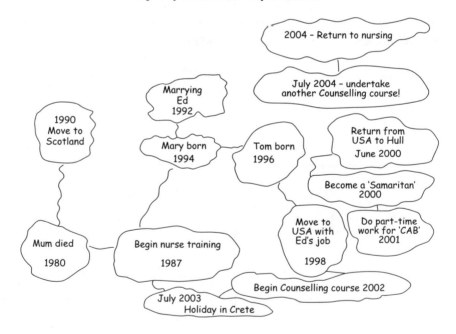

3   Now begin to add branches to your topic as ideas flow into your brain. Don't worry about neat writing or straight lines. In mind mapping it is important to get your thoughts down quickly, before you lose them. If your idea is completely new, and appears to have little connection to anything you have on your paper, create a new branch.

My important life experiences

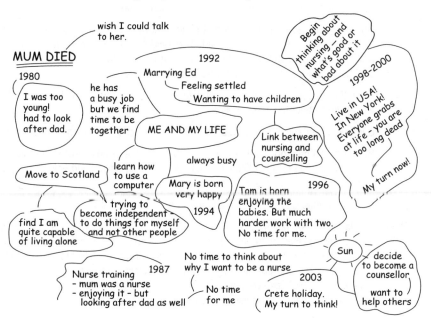

wish I could talk to her.

MUM DIED

1980

I was too young! had to look after dad.

he has a busy job but we find time to be together

1992

Marrying Ed

Feeling settled

Wanting to have children

ME AND MY LIFE

Begin thinking about nursing — and what's good or bad about it

1998-2000

Live in USA! In New York! Everyone grabs at life - you are too long dead

Link between nursing and counselling

My turn now!

Move to Scotland

learn how to use a computer

always busy

Mary is born very happy

1994

Tom is born 1996 enjoying the babies. But much harder work with two. No time for me.

find I am quite capable of living alone

trying to become independent to do things for myself and not other people

Nurse training 1987
- mum was a nurse
- enjoying it - but looking after dad as well

No time to think about why I want to be a nurse

No time for me

2003

Crete holiday. My turn to think!

Sun

decide to become a counsellor

want to help others

---

4   Keep adding details until your thoughts have run dry. Remember to include drawings, and/different shapes and forms so that your mind map looks appealing.

My life experiences

1980   Mum died.
        Was about to leave home for teacher training course – but dad wasn't coping with Mum's death. So I deferred my place and stayed at home to look after him.

1987   Began nurse training. Dad was ill.

1990   Moved to Scotland.
        After dad died I needed to get away. Sold the house and moved somewhere I didn't know anybody. Felt scared.

1992   Married Ed.
        The best thing to happen to me. Settled down for the first time. I was really happy.

1994   Mary was born – she was a brilliant baby.

1996   Tom was born. He cried a lot. I felt depressed a lot of the time. But Ed always there for me.

1998   Ed gets posting to New York. I loved New York. We suddenly had money to do things. Mary caught a bad flu virus. I slept by her bed for 3 nights. She was alright thank goodness The nurse were wonderful.

2000   Came home to Hull. Although it was good to be home I felt a bit lost. For the first time in a very long time I had some time on my hands. I began to get panic attacks and would shout at the kids for no reason and tell Ed I was unhappy.

Got some counselling! I realised that I had not grieved over my mother's death. I had been so busy looking after dad I had 'held it all in' and now I wanted to 'let it all out'. Also I hadn't realised until then that I had been angry and resentful at Dad that I had stayed at home for so long and looked after him.

After this I began to feel better and take control of my life. I decided that I would like to become a counsellor.

2000   Became a Samaritan. Really enjoyed it and found I am good with helping people.

2001   Began part-time work for the Citizens Advice Bureau. I enjoyed this and found that I am not just good at listening, but also at giving advice and helping people to make practical decisions.

2002   Began a Counselling course to help me to develop my skills

2003   Holiday in Crete. Taking time out with Ed was brilliant. It gave me a chance to take stock. My life has been so busy and I have just fallen into things. I realised that although I enjoyed counselling I am very practical. I would like to help people both through enabling them to make decisions, as well as giving practical help. All this made me realise that I was missing nursing! That nursing can offer me the chance to develop my counselling skills alongside.

2004   Enrol on a return to nursing course!

Once you have completed your mind map you can then begin to analyse the information you have included. Look for connections between ideas and information on one end of your piece of paper to another. Now, begin to label common themes and ideas. Look to see if there is anything unusual that you would not have expected to see included. It might be a topic you might want to return to and explore in more depth again.

ACTIVITY 3: goal and action planning

Writing a goal and action plan will help you to identify and plan what you need to complete your profile and set a realistic timescale for completion. Before you start it is worth taking time to think about the purpose of goal and action planning.

Long-term goals. These can cover a variety of topics and include completing your profile, submitting it for academic credit and/or enrolling on a course.

Short-term goals. These are more specific and relate to the things you need to do in order to reach your long-term goals. Usually, they have a clear and contained objective. An example of a short-term goal might be:

Write to manager of care home asking for reference to include in my profile.

Writing down your goals

It is a good idea to write your goals down, as this will help you to make sure you achieve them. Your goals need to be: clearly written and realistic. To say: 'I want the manager of the care home to write about me so I can put it in my profile' is not a goal. To say: 'I want the manager of the care home I worked in between 1997–1998 to write a reference to include in my profile' is.

To help you write a goal and action plan we have included a Goal and Action Plan Form at the back of this chapter. This can be photocopied. However, this is only our idea for what should be included. You might want to design your own form.

ACTIVITY 4: understanding your learning style

We learn in different ways. Some forms of learning might suit some people and not others. Some of us prefer to learn through doing practical tasks whilst others prefer to learn through reflection and analysis. In truth, to learn effectively, we often need to combine practice and theory. Sometimes people feel they are not good at learning and 'it's not for me'. Whereas, it might be that they are using a learning style that is not best for them. Understanding the way you learn, therefore, will help you to make your learning more effective. However, this does not mean that you cannot learn using a style that is not your best. Quite the opposite. Working to improve your learning using a style that is new or difficult can often enable you to deepen and enrich your learning.

There is a vast amount of literature on learning styles. However, it is generally acknowledged that there are four different types of learners:

Activists

Activists prefer new experiences. They are receptive and enthusiastic about new ideas, and get bored doing the same things over and over again. Activists tend to act first and think later. By definition they are active – and therefore do not like situations that require them to be passive. In short, they can also hog the limelight.

Activists learn best
- when they are exposed to new problems, ideas, situations
- working in teams – where they have a clear role
- being thrown in the deep end to solve a problem
- leading a team, etc.

Activists least like learning activities that require them to:
- be methodical and precise
- absorb and analyse data
- listen for too long (e.g. long lectures).

Reflectors

Reflectors like to reflect. They prefer to stand back from an immediate situation and think about it from different perspectives. Reflectors often collect data and think about them. They prefer to observe and to listen to a range of views before coming to any conclusions.

Reflectors learn best:
- in groups (at work or at college)
- in situations where they can review material, and think about what they are learning
- when they are asked to write essays or reports and to analyse data.

Reflectors least like learning activities which require them to:
- take the lead
- role play
- come to a situation without having prepared
- be rushed or exposed to new situations.

Theorists

Theorists are logical people who think problems through in a logical way. They like analysis and tend to be detached and objective about things rather than subjective or emotional. Theorists are usually comfortable using theories and models to explain things. They are less comfortable with creative thinking. They make good researchers!

Theorists learn best:
- in complex situations where they have to use their own skills and knowledge
- in structured situations which are clearly focused
- when they are able to question and think about ideas even if they are not necessarily relevant to their learning needs.

Theorists least like learning activities which require them to:
- show their emotions or feelings
- work in an unstructured way, where there appears to be no purpose
- where they are required to do things that have not been explained.

Pragmatists

Pragmatists like to try things out. They like theories and ideas that have a practical application and can be applied to their work. They are practical people who get frustrated with learning that cannot be applied to their practice

Pragmatists learning best when:
- the learning has practical relevance (e.g. to their work)
- role-playing when they are able to try ideas out in practice
- when they learn things that have clear benefits for practice.

Pragmatists least like learning activities which require them to:
- learn something with little immediate practical benefit
- there are no guidelines on how to do it
- it is all theory.

This activity is adapted from the work of Kolb (1984) and is designed to help you to explore how you learn best.

Read each of the statements below which describe how you learn and if you agree more than you disagree put a tick inside the box. Do not mark the statements where you disagree more than you agree

	a	b	c	d
1	I like to get involved ☐	I like to take my time before acting ☐	I am particular about what I like ☐	I like things to be useful ☐
2	I like to try things out ☐	I like to analyse things and break them into parts ☐	I am open to new experiences ☐	I like to look at all sides of issues ☐
3	I like to watch ☐	I like to follow my feelings ☐	I like to be doing things ☐	I like to think about things ☐
4	I accept people and situations the way they are ☐	I like to be aware of what is around me ☐	I like to evaluate ☐	I like to take risks ☐
5	I have gut feelings and hunches ☐	I have a lot of questions ☐	I am logical ☐	I am hard working and get things done ☐
6	I like concrete things things I can see, feel touch or smell ☐	I like to be active ☐	I like to observe ☐	I like ideas and theories ☐
7	I prefer learning in the here and now ☐	I like to consider and reflect about them ☐	I like to think about the future ☐	I like to see the results of my work ☐
8	I have to try things out for myself ☐	I rely on my own ideas ☐	I rely on my own observations ☐	I rely on feelings ☐
9	I am quiet and reserved ☐	I am energetic and enthusiastic ☐	I tend to reason things out ☐	I am responsible about things ☐

To identify the learning style you prefer to use you will need to use the grid on page 136. Only put down the marks against the numbers in the box. Some numbers (e.g. 1c) are not included in this list. This is intentional.

CE	RO	AC	AE
1A	1B	2B	2A
2C	2D	3D	3C
3B	3A	4C	6B
4A	6C	6D	7D
8D	8C	8B	8A
9B	9A	9C	9D
Calculation 1: Totals			
CE:	RO:	ACı	AE:

These scores can now be plotted on the diagram below:
An analysis of each of the above learning styles is as follows:

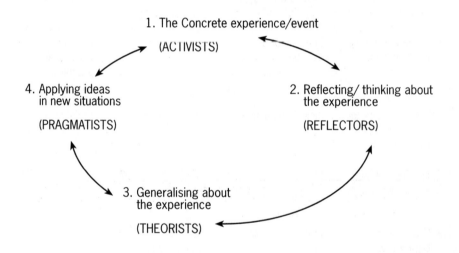

Concrete Experience (Activists)

You prefer being involved in experiences and handling human interactions in a personal way. This learning style emphasises feelings as opposed to thinking; a concern with the uniqueness and complexity of present reality as opposed to theories; these learners prefer intuitive, artistic approaches rather than systematic, scientific problem solving. These learners enjoy and are good at relating to others. They are often good intuitive decision makers and function well in unstructured situations, they relate to people and have an open-minded approach to life.

The characteristics of these people are that they:

- are imaginative, good at generating ideas
- can view situations from different angles
- are open to experience
- recognise problems
- investigate and sense opportunity.

Reflective Observation (Reflectors)

You prefer to focus on understanding the meaning of ideas and situations by observing and describing them. This learning style emphasises understanding as opposed to practical application. These learners are more concerned with what is true, or how things happen, as opposed to what will work. You prefer reflection as opposed to action. These learners prefer intuiting the meaning of situations and ideas and are good at seeing the implications. They look at things from different perspectives and appreciate different points of view. They like to rely on their own thoughts and feelings to form opinions. These people value patience, impartiality and considered, thoughtful judgement.

Abstract Conceptualisation (Theorists)

You prefer to focus on logic, ideas and concepts. You prefer thinking as opposed to feeling, and building general theories, rather than intuitive understanding. These learners prefer a scientific as opposed to an artistic approach to problem solving. These people are good at systematic planning, manipulation of abstract symbols, and analysis. They value precision, and the rigour of analysing ideas.

Active Experimentation (Pragmatists)

These learners focus on actively influencing people and changing situations. You prefer practical application as opposed to reflective understanding. You prefer to deal with what works as opposed to what is absolute truth; the emphasis here is on doing rather than observing. These learners prefer getting things accomplished. They are willing to take some risks in order to achieve their objectives. They also value having an influence on the environment around them. See Kolb, 1984.

Activity 5: PEST analysis

While a SWOT analysis is a useful way of looking at your learning needs from the perspective of your own knowledge and capabilities, it may be useful to look at some of the external factors that may affect you. Health and social care often seem to be in a constant state of reorganisation, as new local and national policies and priorities move the goalposts, and understanding those that affect you can help you to identify your current and future learning needs.

Although it is impossible to see into the future, there are ways minimising the risk that future changes will bring unexpected learning needs or damage your career prospects, and of increasing the chances that you can benefit from these changes. One way is to undertake a PEST analysis. This is similar to a SWOT analysis, except it involves looking at external factors that may influence your profession. Many companies undertake PEST analyses when planning their future business strategies, but the technique is equally useful in analysing trends in health and social care. PEST stands for Political, Economic, Social and Technological factors, all of which can affect the way health and social care are delivered. This means they can also affect you and your career.

Before you conduct a PEST analysis, you should be clear about what you are analysing. You may decide, for example, that you want to work in a particular field such as mental health or children and families, and to analyse that, or you may want to look more generally at influences on health care, social care or both, to help you decide what direction to take. In fact, it can be more useful to conduct a PEST analysis before you conduct a SWOT analysis as it can help you to look at your own situation in relation to the external factors that affect it.

It is impossible to list all the factors you may need to look at in a PEST analysis, as it will depend on what exactly you are analysing, but the following lists should give you some ideas.

Political factors

Current legislation and priorities   These might include, for example, local guidelines on service delivery, national service frameworks, the Care Standards Act, the Mental Health Act, *The NHS Plan* or guidelines issued by the National Institute for Clinical Excellence.

Future legislation and priorites   These might include statements and initiatives from the government, or your own health or local authority, or manifestoes produced locally or nationally by political parties – particularly if an election is due.

Regulatory bodies   These might include a requirement to register, new educational standards or standards governing professional practice.

Funding   This might include the move to integrate health and social care budgets, or extra money being made available to tackle cancer or intermediate care.

Economic factors

The current economic situation   This might include new money being made available for the provision of health and social care, or financial pressures caused by new requirements such as the registration of care homes.

Economic trends   These might include forecasts of an economic downturn that may affect budgets available for service provision.

Organisational priorities   These might include plans for a new multidisciplinary community care team, or to expand an existing service or scale down an existing one due to changing needs in the local population.

Social factors

Lifestyle trends   These might include increasing numbers of people living alone meaning more home care is required, or increasing prevalence of drug use resulting in increased requirements for drug rehabilitation services.

Demographics   These might include the growing number of older people requiring health and social care to maintain their health and independence, or a growing local ethnic minority population with specific needs.

Technological

New technologies and developments   These might include advances in the care of premature babies resulting in increased need for neonatal units, new therapies increasing survival rates in diseases such as cancer or heart disease.

Research funding   These might include funding to investigate the most effective way of providing care or treatment to particular groups, or to find new ways of solving problems.

Information and communication   These might include plans to set up computerised integrated health and social care records accessible by professionals in all settings, or the provision of portable computers for practitioners working in the community.

The factors you need to consider in your PEST analysis will depend on the area you choose to analyse. It may be a good idea to discuss which you should include with a senior colleague or tutor, who may be able to help you to identify those that are relevant to you. They may also be able to help you to identify exactly what you should analyse, depending on your current situation and future ambitions.

Whatever you decide to look at in your PEST analysis, it may help you to identify new avenues that may be open to you in the future, or those which may be closing as a result of changes in care provision.

Goal and action plan form

Name........................... **Date**...................

Goal **Deadline for achieving my goal ...**

Criteria for success
(How will you know when you have
achieved your goal?)

Action plan
(The actions you need to undertake to
achieve your goal)

Summary
(A brief note stating what you have
achieved from the actions taken to
achieve your goal)

Making changes
(Do you need to revise your action
plan in the light of the conclusions
made in your summary?)

REFERENCE

Kolb, D. (1984) *Experiential Learning: Experiences as a Source of Learning and Development*, Englewood Cliffs, NJ: Prentice Hall.

Annotated Bibliography

Profiling documents and texts

Brown, R. A. (1995) *Portfolio Development and Profiling for Nurses* (2nd edn), Central Health Studies Series No. 3 (series editor, John Tingle), Lancaster: Quay Publishing.

This publication offers a well-structured guide to developing your profile, including the collection of material for specific purposes. It provides a good, easy-to-read introduction to the subject.

Churchill Livingstone Professional Portfolio for Nurses, Midwives and Health Visitors (1993), Edinburgh: Churchill Livingstone.

Designed with the user in mind, this personal portfolio offers a lucid and concise framework within which to build a personalised account of your career; past, present and future. The binder is divided into two distinct parts, with labelled dividers for the different sections. Part A focuses on profiles, general and professional education, professional employment and professional development. It provides you with a place to record your personal details, under pre-printed headings, associated with the above. It will be particularly useful in relation to developing your curriculum vitae (CV), applying for a new post, and seeking accreditation of prior learning. Part B helps you to focus on your current and future development, addressing the areas of goal planning and review, critical incident analysis, development of action plans, continuing education activities, and CV writing. This will be particularly useful in relation to performance review, preparation of development plans, and documenting evidence for NMC purposes.

Emap Healthcare Open Learning (1999) *Profile.Pack*, London: Emap Healthcare Open Learning.

The *Profile Pack* enables you to develop and maintain a useful and unique professional portfolio that meets your own needs as well as professional requirements. You can use it for both public and private purposes. It contains a workbook to guide you through the profiling process, with a variety of activities for you to participate in and reflect on; a library binder to store all your work, particularly confidential records; a profile binder that you can use to present work to potential employers or course providers, or records of your professional development; a set of record sheets for you to develop and maintain your profile.

Emap Healthcare Open Learning (2000) *Lifeline Pack*. London: Emap Healthcare Open Learning.

The *Lifeline Pack* can be used in a similar way to a profile, but it focuses on helping you to make decisions about how best to use your skills in the future. Using a combination of self-assessment activities and case studies, it will help you to 'unpack' your current knowledge and experience. Working through the *Lifeline Pack* will build your understanding of modern care provision and allow you to identify career options that will help you achieve your potential. You can use it alongside your profile to make the best use of your learning and to identify future learning that can help you to achieve your ambitions as well as meeting your professional development needs.

Moon, J. (2000) *Reflection in Learning and Professional Development: Theory and Practice*, London: Routledge Falmer.

This book clarifies the background to reflection and reflective practice. It provides a model for reflective practice as well as a wealth of information on the literature of reflection. It also provides practical activities to help people improve their reflection and journal writing skills.

Redmond, B. (2004) *Reflection in Action: Developing Reflective Practice in Health and Social Services*, Aldershot: Ashgate Publishing.

This book outlines a reflective teaching and learning model that can be used by single or multidisciplinary healthcare practitioners. It shows how different models of reflection can be introduced into different levels of training.

White, L. (2000) *Reflection Time: Developing a Reflective Approach to Teaching and Learning*, London: Church House.

This book aims to explain the development of reflective practice. It is aimed primarily at teachers and explains why reflection is a valuable tool for learning and provides activities to help tutors structure reflective sessions.

Study skills

Northedge, A. (2004) *The Good Study Guide*, Milton Keynes: OU Worldwide.

This book is good for students who are re-entering formal learning after a long break and experienced students who need to develop one or more aspects of their study technique. The book is interactive, with activity breaks at regular intervals. Key point summaries are also provided (in a different colour) to help you to focus your mind on your specific learning. In addition to the issues covered in most study skills guides, this book looks at handling numbers confidently. It is designed to meet the needs of social science and humanities students, including adults studying part-time.

Rowntree, D. (1998) *Learn How to Study* (4th edn), London: Time Warner.

This book has been a bestseller since 1970. It has been updated to include the latest research findings related to effective study. It introduces the idea of reflection in the preface. The basic philosophy appears to be the empowerment of students by encouraging the examination of a range of approaches to study, thereby enabling them to utilise the most appropriate technique based upon their personal preference and the purpose of their study. The book is extremely easy to read, with many interactive activities interspersed throughout the theoretical text

Rowntree, D. (1993) *Teach Yourself with Open Learning* (2nd edn), London: Kogan Page.

This lively and engaging book helps learners to make the most of what is available for them in learning. Although the focus is on open learning, the approach is relevant to profile development and reflective practice. The book provides the opportunity to 'dip in' as required and has bold headings and chapter objectives that help you to decide what you want to read. The activities, interspersed throughout the book, provide you with adequate space to note your thoughts. Follow-up activities, which often rely upon interaction with others, provide the opportunity to apply the theory to your practice. Each chapter culminates in a 'reflective activity' that encourages you to sit down and think about your learning.

Career development

Bolles, R. (1998) *What Colour is Your Parachute?*, Enfield, Middlesex: Ten Speed Press.

This book, which is updated annually, is the UK edition of the best-selling US guide to self-analysis and pro-active job-hunting. The British edition comprises the US text with its variety of interactive exercises. The 'pink pages' at the back, which provide a resource directory, is unfortunately heavily influenced by availability within the US. However, the overall system is well tried and tested.

Covey, S. R. (2001) *The 7 Habits of Highly Effective People*, East Roseville, New South Wales, Australia: Simon & Schuster.

This best-selling book helps you to solve both personal and professional problems by adopting a holistic, integrated and principle-centred approach.

It provides many anecdotes and insights into 'effectiveness'. Covey presents a programmed journey for living, with the emphasis on integrity, fairness, honesty and adaptability to change. He asserts that these are essential features if you are to take advantage of the opportunities that change creates. The book is enhanced by the Application Suggestions which are included at the end of each chapter.

Hopson, B. and Scally, M. (2000) *Build Your Own Rainbow: A Workbook for Career and Life Management*, London: Management Books.

This interactive and easy-to-use workbook comprises a number of exercises designed to help you analyse and develop your personal skills, talents and aspirations. It provides the key to a number of essential career development skills, including self-awareness, learning from experience, research skills, goal setting and action planning, decision making and communicating. The exercises in the book encourage you to discover what is important to you about your work, interests and transferable skills. You will be helped to set personal career objectives and make action plans to enable you to take more control of yourself and your life.

Peddlar, M. and Boydell, T. (1999) *Managing Yourself*, London: Lemos & Crane.

This is one of the early books of the *Successful Manager* series. This practical guide contains case studies and useful activities that are designed to help you enhance your practice of self-management, with a view to improving your life and performance at work and elsewhere. The book provides a logical approach, introducing themes, developing them further, and offering an opportunity for in-depth analysis. You are encouraged to use the analysis to make decisions and action plan your life, implement your plan and review the outcomes of your action. This process is achieved in a variety of ways, including questionnaires, case studies to promote thinking, and exercises to improve self-management. The final chapter is blank – apart from the heading – as it is for you to develop your personal plan.

Rouillard, L. (1994) *Goals and Goal Setting*, London: Kogan Page.

The authors consider that this book is unlike many on the subject. It is 'designed to be read with a pencil', with an abundance of activities, exercises, case studies and assessments that require learner participation. The object of the book is to enhance understanding and valuing of personal goals and goal setting. It provides a good, basic introduction to the level of achievement which goal setting can accomplish. The book could be used in many ways, including individual study, workshops and seminars, and informal study groups.

Wright, B. (1996) *Which Way Now? How to Plan and Develop a Successful Career*, London: Piatkus.

This book claims to be a self-investor's guide to life, work and career – full of good sense, help and pragmatism. It suggests ways in which you can be in control of your future, shows how to set short- and long-term goals, demonstrates how to match your skills and values with the right jobs, and shows how to use creative thinking to develop your career. Phase 1 explores aspects of self-knowledge. Phase 2 focuses on exploring your options, including going it alone. Phase 3 concentrates on action planning and basic communication skills, personal presentation and written communication skills. Phase 4 concludes with career monitoring and career maintenance.

Ways of learning

Boud, D., Cohen, R. and Walker, D. (eds) (1993) *Using Experience for Learning*, Buckingham: OU Press.

This book addresses the struggle of trying to make sense of learning from experience. It explores concepts such as: What are the key ideas that underpin 'learning from experience'? How do we learn from experience? How does context and purpose influence learning? How does experience impact on individual and group learning? How can we help others to learn from their experience? This book addresses the use of experiential learning in the contexts of informal and formal learning. It does not offer simple strategies of how to make it work, but explores the underpinning philosophy of experiential learning.

Boud, D., Keogh, R. and Walker, D. (1985) *Reflection: Turning Experience into Learning*, London: Kogan Page.

This book synthesises the many theoretical insights, from across a variety of fields, about the potential of reflection. Furthermore, these insights are illuminated with recent practical examples. Thus, the relation of theory to practice (and vice versa) is well illustrated. The book contains an examination of the nature of reflection and its role in the learning process. It focuses on the place of writing, discussion and conversation in reflection.

Brookfield, S. D. (1991) *Developing Critical Thinkers: Challenging Adults to Explore Alternative Ways of Thinking and Acting*, Chichester: Jossey-Bass Wiley.

This book aims to introduce readers to critical thinking. The central theme is the need to make the connection between the reader's private life and the broader social forces. It examines the methods that can be used by those seeking to introduce the concept of critical thinking to others. It also explores the opportunities for developing critical thinking in four specific areas: intimate relationships; workplace; political involvement; and the mass media. The book is divided into three sections: the concept of critical thinking; helping people to become critical thinkers; and opportunities for developing critical thinking in specific contexts. The book is well illustrated with case studies and exercises, and also includes an extensive reference list.

Downs, S. (1995) *Learning at Work*, London: Kogan Page.

This lively, easy-to-use book is designed to help manager, trainer and learner to recognise and overcome obstacles to learning. It provides a practical guide to understanding and practising the concepts that help people learn. The book is interspersed throughout with cartoons and checklists to amplify its message. It also points out the myths, pitfalls and blockages that stand in the way of successful learning. The book is divided into seven sections: sections 1 and 2 explore beliefs about learning; section 3 concentrates upon designing training material for learning; section 4 focuses on developing training material to develop understanding; section 5 discusses developing learning through group involvement; section 6 provides an example of a workshop ('Working safely in times of change'); and section 7 suggests some criteria to use when reviewing training materials.

Evans, N. (1994) *Experiential Learning for All*, Guildford and King's Lynn: Cassel Education.

This book offers a snapshot portrayal of experiential learning in the various contexts in which it has developed over the last decade. Each chapter provides a different focus, and in doing so draws on the experience of practitioners from many fields of education. Assessment of prior experiential learning is defined and considered in the contexts of higher education, further education, adult education, the professions, teacher education, employment and unemployment, assessment, staff development and, finally, international developments. The concluding chapter projects the future of the assessment of experiential learning.

Marshall, L. and Rowland, F. (2001) *A Guide to Learning Independently* (2nd edn), Harlow: Prentice Hall.

This book offers a comprehensive range of techniques to help you succeed in education. It emphasises the importance of identifying your own learning needs and the techniques that best suit you. This latest edition includes new study techniques and advice based on current learning theory and research. Updated topics include correct referencing and the use of computers in tasks such as essay writing. The diverse cultural background of students is acknowledged. This is a book for a wide range of students and teachers, engaged in both practical and theoretical courses and in science and humanities. Although there is a degree of interactivity, it is not as obvious as for many other study skills workbooks.

McNiff, J. and Whitehead, N. (1992) *Teaching as Learning: An Action Research Approach*, London: Routledge.

This book presents the authors' account of their own work and professional development. The study is based on the hypothesis that educational knowledge is created by individuals at work, rather than by researchers in institutions of higher education. The aim of this book is to encourage practitioners to make sense of their own practice, while evaluating the contributions of other thinkers. This fascinating and personal book works with case studies of actual practice. The authors use the familiar action research paradigm of identifying a problem; imagining, implementing and evaluating a solution; and modifying practice in the light of that evaluation. They give practical advice that will aid the professional development of the researcher and practitioner alike, and conclude that the best teaching is done by those who want to learn and can show others how to be open to their own processes in self-development.

Palmer, A., Burns, S. and Bulman, C. (eds) (2004) *Reflective Practice in Nursing: The Growth of the Professional Practitioner*, London: Blackwell Scientific.

This book provides an easy-to-read resource for nurse practitioners and educationalists who wish to explore the area of reflective practice in nursing. Its contributors come from a wide range of backgrounds, but are all actively engaged in the development of reflective practice. The book takes you through the various stages of reflection and encourages you to to make more sense of clinical practice. There is no requirement to read the book from cover to cover as its style enables you to dip into the aspect in which you are most interested. This aspect might be the nature and theories of reflective learning, the facilitation and assessment of reflective learning, or your personal experience, for example.

Weil, S. and McGill, I. (eds) (1989) *Making Sense of Experiential Learning*, Buckingham: OU Press.

This book explores the multiplicity of meanings and practices associated with experiential learning in an international context. The editors have identified four discrete perspectives from amongst the contributors. These different perspectives are identified as 'villages', which contribute towards the 'global village'. The book illustrates the complexities of experiential learning and challenges readers to use the benefits of experiential learning in their own lives.

Whittaker, P. (1996) *Managing to Learn*, London: Cassell.

This readable, well-researched book is one of the Cassell series of *Pastoral Care and Personal and Social Education*. The premise for the book is that the ability to facilitate learning is one of the most awesome tasks that a teacher confronts. It helps teachers to organise learning in such a way that an individual student's potential is released and capitalised upon, whilst societal needs are also met. The author's main theme is that the student requires instruction for knowledge and practice, alongside the opportunity to develop the skills to reflect deliberately upon the process of learning itself. Although this book is apparently written for school teachers, the content is applicable to adult education. Section 1 – Learners and Learning – draws on the work of Knowles, Freire and Boud and Walker, for example. Section 2 – Teachers and Teaching – reviews the role of the teacher as both a manager and a leader, providing some frameworks to work within. Section 3 – Classrooms and Schools – is applicable to any learning organisation. Section 4 – The A–Z of Learning – provides definitive paragraphs based around terminology on topics such as accountability, beliefs, communication and emotion.

Index

Notes: f = figure; n = note; t = table; **bold** extended discussion or heading emphasised in main text

accommodators (learning type)   **112**
accreditation   xvi, 25, 26, 71, 94–5, 99, 142
  claiming credit for prior learning (four
      stages)   **102–6**
  continuing professional development   **96**
  portfolios   **101–7**
  towards a definition   **95**
Accreditation of Prior Experiential Learning
    (APEL)   18, 28, **36**, 63, 102–3, 105–6
Accreditation of Prior Learning (APL)   **36**
action plans   *see* goal and action plans
activities
  lifeline   53–4
  professional values   54–5
  useful 145
activists (type of learner)   **133**, 136f, **136–7**
admiration (professional value)   55
adult education   xiv, **6–7**, 46, 99, 147, 149
  'adult learning'   xvi, 113
  'evening classes'   25
  'further education'   12, 46, 147
Advanced Vocational Certificate in Education
    (AVCE)   101t
advising (facilitation skill)   **116**
aesthetics   88, 89
age   54, 97, 114
anger   84
APEL   *see* Accreditation of Prior Experiential
    Learning
apprenticeship systems   31
art portfolios   28
articles (written)   71, 73, 74, 104
aspirations   73, 74, 145
assessing (facilitation skill)   **116**
assimilators (learning type)   **112**
AVCE *see* Advanced Vocational Certificate in
    Education
awarding bodies   38, **99–100**, **107**
awards   *see* post-qualifying awards

Basic Skills   28
Belenky, M., *et al.* (1986)   46, 47
  Clinchy, B.   47
  Goldberger, N.   47
  Taroule, J.   47
beliefs   64, 65f, 79, 114, 149
benchmarking   18, 70
best practice   17
bias-avoidance   104
bibliography (annotated)   xiv, **142–9**
  career development   144–6
  interactivity   143, 144, 148
  profiling documents and texts   142–3
  reflective practice   76, 88, 143, 144, 146,
      148
  study skills   143–4
  ways of learning   146–9

biography   40
Blunkett, D.   23–4
Bolles, R.   144
Boud, D.   33, **146**, 149
Boud, D., *et al.* (1985)   33, 36, 76, 92, 122,
      124, **146**
  Keogh, R.   36, 92, 124, **146**
  Walker, D.   36, 92, 124, **146**
boundaries
  academic versus professional   31–2
  professional and service   18, 27
Boyd, E. M.   80
Boydell, T.   145
Brookfield, S. D.   **146–7**
Brown, R. A.   28–9, 142
Build your own Rainbow (Hopson and Scally,
      2000)   145
Bulman, C.   148
Burns, S.   148
Business and Technical Education Council
    (BTEC)   107
Buzan, T.   130

cadet schemes   **27**
campaigns   73
cancer   138, 139
care   10, 13–14
  domiciliary   17
care in the community   64
care homes (registration)   138
care plans   72
Care Standards Act (2000)   19, 96, 138
Care Trusts   16
careers   18, 52, 54, 91, 137
  see continuing professional development
carers/caring   9, 19, 51, 127
Carper, B.   88
  'patterns of knowing'   88–9
case studies   82, 145, 147
Central Council for Education and Training in
    Social Work (CCETSW)   22
certificates of attendance   104
child care   17
child-raising   50, 52, 65f, 110, 126
Chinese proverb   49
choice   38, 89
*Churchill Livingstone Professional Portfolio for
    Nurses, Midwives and Health Visitors*
    (1993)   142
City and Guilds   107
Clarke, B.   77
clients   9, 17, 24, 25, 27, 29, 32, 33, 89, 97
Clinchy, B.   47
clinical governance   13
clinical supervision   12, 77
Code of Practice for Social Care Workers   19
Cohen R.   **146**

colleagues   20, 64, 112, 122
   peers   47
   protection   83, 84–5
   senior   47, 139
colour   130
Commission for Health Improvement   13
communication   25, 30, 40, 54, 62–3, 64, 73,
   74, 91, 139, 145, 149
   'key skill'   35, 99
   oral   69
   written   69
communication skills   146
community care   138
community groups   51
competence   95, 97–8, 98t, 100t, 101, 102,
   106, 110, 119
competence statements   **66–70**
competencies   59, 63, 71, 72, 74
computers   118, 122, 139, 148
   computer packages   29, 71, 103
concepts   40, 41, 65f, 130, 137
conceptualisation   63, **111**, 112
conferences   21
   seminars   51, 122
   workshops   xiii, 73, 104, 147
confidence   30, 50, 51, 81, 87, 113–14, 116,
   118, 128
confidentiality   5–6, 9, 13, 47, 71, **83–5**, 143
   protection of diarist   83–4
   protection of patients and colleagues   83,
   84–5
connections   41, 42, 49, **63–6**, 119, 128,
   130, 132
   Kolb's learning cycle (adapted)   109f, **111**
context   77, 84–5
continuing professional development (CPD)
   xiii, 1, 2, 3, 10, 31, 41
   accreditation (national schemes)   **96**
   annotated bibliography   **144–6**
   core principles   27
   initiatives   27–8
   key characteristics   4
   lifelong learning   13–14
   multidisciplinary teams   **34**
   'professional development'   6, 9, 24, 30,
   38–9, 40, 44, **52–5**, 63, 73, 81, 108,
   116–17
   programmes   8
   social care context   **21–2**
   terminology   **26–8**
   useful points to remember   3
   see also lifelong learning
*Continuing Professional Development: Quality
   in the NHS* (1999)   27
conventional wisdom   111
convergers (learning type)   **112**
courses   5, 11, 14, 39, 52, 60, 71, 104
   applications   55–6
   practical and theoretical   148
   short   47, 126
   taught   21, 46, 122
Covey, S. R.   144–5
CPD *see* continuing professional development
craft guilds   31
Credit Accumulation and Transfer Scheme
   (CATS)   22, 106

Credit Framework (higher education)   96
credit frameworks   **35**
critical incident analysis   (Flanagan)   86,
   142
critical incidents   11, 86, 90, 91
cross-referencing   48, **72–3**
culture   24, 49, 148
curricula   46, 104
curriculum vitae (CV)   10–11, 40, 142

data   133
decision-making   14, 16, 64, 70, 77, 95, 112,
   121, 145
   professional value   54
demographics/demography   128, 139
Department of Education and Employment
   17, 24
Department for Education and Skills   13,
   24–5
Department of Health   17, 19, 27, 28
dependence   24, 117, 122
*Developing Critical Thinking: Challenging
   Adults to Explore Alternative Ways of
   Thinking and Acting* (Brookfield, 1991)
   146–7
development process   61f
Dewey, J.   30–1, 76
diagrams   83, 87
disciplinary committees   6
discussion   32, 46, 81, 109, 146
divergers (learning type)   **112**
doctors   19
Downs, S.   147
drawings   29, 72, 83, 104
drugs (narcotics)   17, 138

economic trends   138
Edexcel   107
education   10, 24, 25, 40, 142, 147
   formal   31, 62
   practice-based   32
education system   49
educational
   activities   51
   counselling (facilitation skill)   **116**
   institutions   xv, 8
   needs   48, 74
   programmes   xvi, **13**, 94, 103
elderly people   64
elections   138
Emap Healthcare Open Learning (EHOL)   8,
   81, 142–3
emotions   31, 123,   134, 149
empirics   88, 89
employers   19, 30, 44, 96, 99
employment   40, 109, 142, 147
enabling (facilitation skill)   **115–16**
England   17, 19
English National Board for Nursing and
   Midwifery (ENB)   4, 10, 26
essays   65, 71, 148
ethics   21, 65, 66, 88, 89
evaluation ('summative' and 'formative')
   124
Evans, N.   147
events   50

evidence   95, 101–2, **103–5**, 142
   direct   **103–4**
   indirect   **104**
evidence-based practice   **18**
examinations   45
exercises   41, 145, 147
expectations   24
experience   12, 14, 27, 33, 34, 37, 38, 41, 45,
      48, **49–52**, 53, 59, 60, 62, 64, 65f, 70,
      71, 73, 74, 77, 81, 82, 89, 94, 95, 104,
      113–14, 118–19, 123
   documenting   60f
   Kolb's learning cycle (adapted)   109f, **110**
   learning from   **108–12**
   life   130–2
   new   133
   personal   126
   professional   126
   reviewed to date   **8**
   significant   61
   systematic reflection   **102–3**
Experiential Learning for All (Evans, 1994)
      147
experiential learning   78, 80, **108–12**, 113,
      145–9
   basic principles   31
   'making sense of ourselves in relation to
      world'   32
   'not merely theory but practice'   31
   terminology   **30–2**
   see also learning
experiential processes   xiv
experimentation   49, 65, 112
   Kolb's learning cycle (adapted)   109f, **111**
external verifiers   106

facilitation   **108–24**, 148
   evaluation   123–4
   ground rules   122–3
   learning environment   122
   planning the profile   118–22
   progress chasing   123
   questions   124
   taking responsibility   117–18, 123
facilitation skills   xvi, **115–17**
   advising   116
   assessing   116
   educational counselling   116
   enabling   115–16
   informing   116–17
facilitators   7, 90, **113**
   first task   115
   role   **121–2**
fairness   145
Fales, A. W.   80
family   25, 47, 53, 95, 109, 118, 121
feelings   45, 46, 81, 88, 134, 136
   positive and negative   87
   private record   48
FHE Curriculum Development Project   66
Flanagan, J. C.   86
Foundation Degrees   28
freedom to learn (Boud *et al.*)   122
Freire, P.   149
friends   25, 47, 90, 118, 121, 122
fund-raising   51

funding   14, 21, 138

gaps   17
General Certificate of Education: Advanced
      Level   45, 100t, 101t
General Certificate of Secondary Education
      (GCSE)   100t, 101t
General National Vocational Qualification
      (GNVQ)   100t
General Social Care Council (2001–)   **19**, 96
Gibbs, L.   18
Gibbs' reflective cycle   78, 79f
global village   149
Goal and Action Plan Form   140
goal and action plans   **9**, 20, 45, 59, 60, 82,
      120–1, 125, 126, 132–3, 142, 145, 146
   long-term/short-term   132
Goals and Goal-Setting (Rouillard, 1994)
      145
Goldberger, N.   47
Good Study Guide (Northedge, 2004)   143–4
Government (UK)   13, 24, 35, 97, 138
government policy   128
   terminology   23
graphs   104
group involvement   147
Guernsey: Institute of Health Studies   9
Guide to Learning Independently (Marshall and
      Rowland, 2001)   147–8
guidelines   41, 70, 134

HCA Profile: Personal Development Pack
      (2001)   7–8
health authorities   138
health care   xiv, 21, 94, 127, 139
   advances   128
   delivery   24
   PEST analysis   137, 138
health care assistants   xiii, 1, 7, 8, 9
health care practitioners/professionals
   lifelong learning   **13–14**
   single- or multi-disciplinary   143
health care staff   24, 25, 26, 27
Health and Social Care Occupational
      Standards   97
health technologies   24–5
health trusts   14
health visitors/visiting   xiii, 1, 2, 4, 7, 38, 81
   PREP standards   3
heart disease   139
helping clients (professional value)   54
higher education   **6–7**, 18, **34**, 99, 147, 148
Hinman, J.   66
hobbies   51, 53, 127
Hoggart, R.   117
holidays   58
Hollingsworth, M.   66
Holm, D.   88
home care   138
honesty   123, 145
Hopson, B.   145
hospitals   14
housing   17
Hudek, K.   xii
Hull, C.   xiv
human interaction   136

human rights   21
humanities   148
Hume, H.   xii

ideas   63, 64, 65f, 66, 79, 111, 127, 130, 132, 134, 137
   new   40, 133
identity   49
individual performance review (IPR)   10, 11
inductive reasoning   112
industrial revolution   31
influence/s   53, 137
information   **45**, 132, 139
   extraction   66
   presentation   66
information management   69
'information processors'   79
information technology
   'key skill'   35, 99
informing (facilitation skill)   **116–17**
institutions   70
integrity   145
interests   53, 54
interpretation   95
interviews   65f, 106

James, C. R.   xii, 77
job applications   **10–11**, 40, 55–6, 58
job interviews   8, 11
job role: influence on learning type (Kolb)   112
job security (professional value)   54
job-hunting   144
job-task diversity (professional value)   54
Johns, C.   80, 85, 88, 89, 90
journals (academic)   21, 121

Keeton, M.   78
Kelly, J.   77
Keogh, R.   36, 92, 124, **146**
key skills   **35–6, 99**
   listed   99
   website   99
knowledge   14, 17, 18, 26, 34, 39, 45, 46, 52, 55, 59, 61–5, 71, 73, 74, 94, 95, 96, 99–100t, 102, 103, 105, 106, 113, 118, 127, 134
   analysis   **68**, 70
   application   **68, 69**, 70
   challenges   114
   four areas needed by nurses and midwives (Carper)   88–9
   integration   112
   interpretation   **67**, 70
   interpretation and application   27
   personal   88–9
   professional   77, 80, 81
   standards   8
   synthesis   **68–9**, 70
   tacit   77
   transferability   43
   understanding   67, 68
knowledge base   77, 87, 91
Knowles, M.   108, 149
Kolb, D.   31, 109, 134
   learning types   111–12

relationship between thinking and experience   31
Kolb's learning cycle   31, 78f, 78, 79, 109f, 110
L'Aiguille, Y.   85
language   41, 42
law courts   6
Learn How to Study (Rowntree, 1998)   144
learners   147
   independence   118
learning   33, 38, 39, 41, 42, 45, 46, 52, **60–1**, 70, 71, 89, 101, 116, 119
   A–Z   149
   affective (subjective)   31
   annotated bibliography   **146–9**
   articulation   **62–3**
   'banking concept'   109–10
   blocks/obstacles   **113–15**, 128, 147
   cognitive (factual)   31
   content   113
   'conversion' of reflection into   90–1
   effectiveness   **xvi, 94–107**
   flexible approaches   94–5
   focus for organising   **11–12**
   formal   43, 82, 94, 108, 146
   identification   **73**
   informal   43, 82, 94, 102, 109, 146
   knowledge   **67–9**
   level/standard   **62**, 105, 106
   method   66
   nature   66
   passive   109–10
   producing competence statements   **66–70**
   professional values   54
   recognition (identification)   **62**
   reflection and   **78–80**
   significant   **61–6, 103**
   testing   **63–6**
   theory and practice   110, 111
   under-utilised   109
   ways   **146–9**
   see also experiential learning
learning (prior): claiming credit   **12–13, 102–6**
   stage 1: systematic reflection on experience   102–3
   stage 2: identification of significant learning   103
   stage 3: identification of evidence to support claims   103–5
   stage 4: submission of profile for formal assessment   105–6
Learning Age (Green Paper, 1998)   24
learning contracts   **119–21**, 123
   action plan   120–1
   fundamental questions   119–20
   goals and criteria for success   120
learning cycles   32, 65f, **109–11**
learning disability   17
learning environment   **57–8**, 116, **122**
Learning from Experience Trust   66
learning how to learn ('key skill')   99
learning needs   7, 116, 147
   identification   xv
learning opportunities   61, 90, 116

learning outcomes 63, 95
  terminology **33–4**
learning process 113, 146
  four stages 49
learning skills **69–70**
learning styles **111–12**, 125, **133–7**
  activists 133, 136f, 136–7
  pragmatists 134, 136f, 137
  reflectors 133–4, 136f, 137
  theorists 134, 136f, 137
learning theories 108
learning types (Kolb) 111–12
  accommodators **112**
  assimilators **112**
  convergers **112**
  divergers **112**
  influence of current job role 112
Learning at Work (Downs, 1995) 147
lectures 51, 122
legislation 138
leisure 54, 109
libraries 47, 118–19, 122
life
  'flowing process' 117–18
  home/work balance 52–3
Lifeline Pack (Emap Healthcare Open
    Learning, 2000) 142
lifelines 50, 53–4
lifelong learning **13–14, 18**, 19, 20, 100
  formal and informal 25
  fruits **26**
  individual needs 25
  initiatives 27–8
  'key to prosperity' 23
  profile approach 27
  terminology **23–6**
  see also continuing professional development
Lifelong Learning (website) 24
lifestyle 24, 54, 138
listening, active 115–16
literacy 28
literature
  learning from reflection 90–1
  learning styles 133
  structures for reflection 87
litigation 6
local authorities 138
logic 137
London University: Goldsmiths College 37
Long-Term Care Charter 16
Lucas, P. 80, 91

Making Sense of Experiential Learning (Weil
    and McGill, 1989) 148–9
management 112
  junior/senior 98
  professional value 55
management development
  social care 17
managers 17, 147
Managing to Learn (Whittaker, 1996) 149
Managing Yourself (Peddlar and Boydell, 1999)
    145
market forces xv, **7–9**
market value 95
Marshall, L. 147–8

mass media 147
McGill, I. 148–9
McNiff, J. 148
memory 50, 114
mental health 17
Mental Health Act 138
Mezirow, J. 110–11
midwifery xiv, 2, 5, 76, 114
  PREP standards 3
midwives xiii, 1, 2–3, 4, 6, 7, 10, 12, 38, 80,
    81
  'Rule 37' 3
mind-mapping 125, **130–2**
Modern Apprenticeships (MAs) 28
*Modernising Social Care Workforce: First
    National Training Strategy for England*
    (2000) 17
Modernising Social Services (White Paper,
    1998)
  implications for social care staff 16–17
modules 33
money (professional value) 54
monitoring 18
moods 50
Moon, J. 143
musical score 103

National Boards 3
  'no longer exist' 4
National Care Standards Commission 96
National Committee of Inquiry into Higher
    Education 34
National Council for Vocational Qualifications
    (NCVQ, 1986–) 97
National Credit Framework 99, 99–100t
National Health Service (NHS) 24–5
  staff 20, 27, 28
National Health Service learning accounts
    (LAs) **27–8**
National Health Service Plan (White Paper,
    2000) 16, 19, 24, 27–8, 138
National Health Service (NHS) Trusts 16
National Institute for Clinical Excellence
    13–14, 138
National Learning and Skills Council (LSC),
    35
National Occupational and Service Standards
    17
National Occupational Standards for Social
    Care (NOSs, 2002–) 19, **96–7**, 106
National Open College Network (NOCN)
    99, 100
National Qualifications Framework (NQF,
    2004–) **100–1**
  aims 35
  essential features 35
  website 101
National Training Strategy 17–18
  aim (social care staff) 18
National Vocational Qualifications (NVQs)
    xiii, 28, 96, **97–8**, 102, 106
  courses 1
  equivalences with OCN **100**
  framework 98t
  health care assistants 1
  historical context 97

National Vocational Qualifications – *continued*
    levels 98t
    National Qualifications Framework
        101t
    students 5
    training 9, 10
networks
    local or regional 21
newspapers 121
NMC *see* Nursing and Midwifery Council
NOCN (National Open College Network)
    99, 100
Nonconformist chapel tradition 117
Northedge, A. 143–4
notebooks 8
Notification of Practice form 3
NQF, *see* National Qualifications Framework
numeracy 28
    'key skill' 99
nurse practitioners 148
nurses xiii, 1, 2–3, 4, 6, 7, 10, 12, 19, 21, 38,
    80, 81, 89, 90
nursing xiv, 2, 5, 76, 87, 114
    PREP standards 3, 4
nursing conferences xiii
nursing curricula
    'central theme' 76–7
Nursing and Midwifery Council (NMC,
    2002–) 3, 4, 5, 9, 44, 77, 90, 142
    address 10
    confidentiality of profiles 84
    requirements for profiling and reflection
        82
    website 8, 10
nursing skills 78
NVQs *see* National Vocational Qualifications

objectivity 134
occupational standards 102
occupations 98
Open College Network (OCN) 96
    credits **99–100**
    equivalences with NVQs **100**
Open University 51
organisational priorities 138
organisations 20

painting 50, 104
Palmer, A. 148
partnership working 18
Pastoral Care and Personal and Social Education
    (Cassell series) 149
patients 9, 13, 17, 18, 24, 25, 27, 29, 32, 33,
    89, 97
    protection 83, 84
patronage 117
Peddlar, M. 145
performance 8, 82, 97, 145
personal development **52–5**, 113
    planning **34**
    website 34
personal goals/objectives 69
    identification **11**
    see also goal and action plans
personal professional portfolios 1, 2–3, 5, 7
    'no approved format' 4

    see also profiles
personal professional profile 10, 81–2
perspective transformation (Mezirow) 110
PEST (Political, Economic, Social,
    Technological) analysis 125, **137–9**
photographs 50, 71, 73, 104
physical changes 50
pictures 73, 83, 87, 130
Piercy, M. 46
place (reflective diary) **85–6**
poems 71
politics 51, 138, 147
portfolio development **18**
Portfolio Development and Profiling for Nurses
    (Brown, 1995) 142
portfolios xiii, 2, 4, 34, 62
    accreditation **101–7**
    content requirements 9
    relevance and quality 28
    terminological 'confusion' 28
    terminology **28–30**
    types 29f
    usage xiv, 5, 30
    volume 28
post-qualifying awards 33, 71, 104
    framework 'under review' 22
    listed 21
Post-Qualifying Training 21
Post-Registration Education and Practice
    (PREP) 1, 2, 4, 77
    CPD standard **2**, 9
    implementation 81–2
    practice standard **2**
    requirements **10**
    summary forms 3
power relationships 111
practice 32, 43, 81, 83, 133, 146, 148
    clinical 104
    evidence-based 32–3
    improvement 80
    learning from 12
    lifelong learning 13–14
    role of reflection **77**
    standards 8
    updating 21, 25
practices 65
practitioners 147
pragmatists (type of learner) **134**, 136f, **137**
PREP *see* Post-Registration Education and
    Practice
PREP Handbook (2002) 3, 10, 84, 90
    framework of questions 82
preparation (of profile) **55–8**
    environment 57–8
    time management 55–7
presentation 70, 73
Price, J. xii
private sector 16, 27
problem-solving 14, 69, 77, 109, 112, 136, 137
    'key skill' 36, 99
    personal and professional 144–5
professional:
    bodies 8, 44
    education 4
    knowledge 6
    record 47

professional conduct cases 6
Professional Profile Folder 5
professionals 90
    behaviour 80–1
    health and social care xiii–xv
professions 147
    characteristics 77
profile classes 37
Profile Pack (1994) 8, 81
Profile Pack (Emap Healthcare Open Learning,
    1999) 143
profile process 38, 65f, 73
profile-construction **70–5**
    appendices 73, 74
    bibliography of publications 73
    contents 71–2
    desirable characteristics 70
    organisation 72–3
    references and testimonials 73
    sample framework 74
    samples from reflective diary 73
    samples of work 73
    writing skills 74–5
profiles xiii, 4, 27, 33, 34
    accreditation **101–7**
    advice and guidance 7, 116
    applications 7
    assessment criteria 105
    benefits 20
    bibliography (annotated) **142–9**
    comments 37
    common questions xiii–xiv
    completion time **44**
    compulsory element of professional
        development 38
    concise and direct 45
    creation (getting started) **xv, 48–75**
    deadlines for completion 44, 119, 123,
        140
    evidence provided 45
    facilitation **xvi, 108–24**
    facilitator's role **121–2**
    'further resources' **xvi, 125–41**
    gaps **45–6**
    help sources **46–7**
    information to be included **45**
    learning level (standard and quality) **44**
    ownership **44**, 116, 117, 121
    planning **118–22**
    private section 40, 53, 71, 143
    professional requirement xiii, 1, 2, 3, 38,
        113
    public record 40–1, 84, 143
    purpose **38–9, 40**
    ready-made/commercially-produced 5,
        7–8, **39–43**
    ready-made versus self-developed 8
    reflection and 81–2
    reflective practice **xv, 76–93**
    reviewing experience to date **8**
    self-appraisal **8–9**
    setting goals and action plans **9**
    strengths and weaknesses (personal) 40
    taking responsibility **117–18**, 119, 121,
        123
    terminological 'confusion' 28

terminology **28–30**
themes and questions **xv, 37–47**
'three broad steps' **8–9**
two sections 9
usage xiv, 5, 30
use as learning tool 31
uses within health care **10–14**
'well worth the effort' 41
profiles: creation (getting started) **xv,
    48–75**
    case studies 50–1, 64
    deadlines 58
    developing a structure 58–60
    identifying significant learning 61–6
    preparation 55–8
    proving what you know and can do
        66–70
    real reasons 50, 51, 52
    reflecting on past learning 60–1
    taking stock 49–58
profiles: purchased **39–43**
    accessibility **41**
    aims and criteria 39
    binders 42, 143
    content **41–2**, 43
    cost **43**
    design and layout **42–3**
    dividers 42
    forms 42
    private record: communicating with yourself
        40
    public record: communicating with others
        40–1
    purpose **40**
    softest option (to be avoided) 41
    workbooks 42–3, 143, 148
profiles: uses within health care **10–13**
    achieving credit as part of a prior learning
        claim 12–13
    assessment for an educational programme
        13
    focus for organising your own learning
        11–12
    identifying personal goals 11
    job applications 10–11
    PREP requirements 10
    supporting learning from practice and
        clinical supervision 12
    tool for reflective practice 12
Profiles and Portfolios (second edition)
    aims xiv
    authorial backgrounds xiv
    contents **xv–xvi**
    first edition xiii
    revision and updating xiii
    use xiv
profiles and portfolios: health care context
    xv, 1–15
    adult and higher education 6–7
    influences 2
    lifelong learning 13–14
    market forces xv, 7–9
    practical issues xiii, xiv–xv
    reflective practice xv, 5–6
    statutory bodies xv, 2–5
    uses within health care 10–13

profiles and portfolios: social care context **xv, 16–22**
  continuing professional development 21–2
  evidence-based practice 18
  lifelong learning 18
  portfolio development 18
  standards for social care 19–21
profiling xiii, xiv, xv, 18, 25–6
  importance 29–30
  reflective practice (two elements) 33
  short courses 47
  three steps 82
profiling documents (annotated bibliography) **142–3**
progress files (two elements) **34**
projects 51
promotion (professional value) 54
public sector 27
publishing xiv

qualifications 13, 19, 21, 28, 29, 33, 40, 43, 52, 74, 95, 126, 128
Qualifications and Curriculum Authority (QCA) 19, 35, 106
qualities 61, 62
quality assurance 17
quality of service 97
questionnaires 145

reading 51
real-life situations 111
received wisdom 114
recognition
  professional value 54
  public 72
recruitment and retention 17
Redfern, L. xiv
Redmond, B. 143
referees 48
references 59, 73, 104, 116
reflection **xv**, 4, 5, 30, 33, 41, **49–52**, 53, **60–1**, 62, 64, 65f, 74, **76–93**, **102–3**, 112, 123, 144, 146
  alternative choices 88
  bibliography (annotated) 143
  confidentiality 83–5
  conversion' into learning 90–1
  definitions 80–1, 91
  elements (Mezirow) 110–11
  five main steps 85–91
  fruits 81
  ideas for further work **91–2**
  individual or group work **90**
  Kolb's learning cycle (adapted) 109f, **110–11**
  learning 78–80
  profiles 81–2
  role in professional practice 77
  series of questions 87, 88
  structured (model) 89
  structures **87–90**
  terminology **32–3**
  two types (Schon) 77
  writing 82–3
Reflection: Turning Experience into Learning (Boud, Keogh and Walker, 1985) 146

reflection-in-action (Schon) 77
reflection-on-action (Schon) 77, 82, 85
Reflection in Action: Developing Reflective Practice in Health and Social Services (Redmond, 2004) 143
Reflection in Learning and Professional Development: Theory and Practice (Moon, 2000) 143
Reflection Time (White, 2000) 143
reflective diary/journal 5–6, 45, 59, 60, 62, 73, 75, 81, 115, 121
  avoidance of trivia 83
  choice of situation or event 86–7
  confidentiality 83–5
  critical reflection on situation or event 87–90
  details of situation 86–7
  experimentation 83
  five main steps **85–91**
  follow-up actions 90–1
  honesty 83–4
  identification of areas of learning 90–1
  'meant to be a workbook' 83
  motivation and commitment 86
  perseverance 83
  positive approach 83
  'private section' 6
  re-evaluation 91
  self-censorship 84
  spontaneity 83–4
  'things of significance' 83
  time and place 85–6
  tips 83
  ways other than writing 83
reflective learner, autonomous 55
reflective practice xiv, **xv**, **5–6**, 12, 26, 30, 32, **76–93**, 144, 148
  'central theme' of nursing curricula 76–7
  definitions 80–1
Reflective Practice in Nursing: Growth of Professional Practitioner (Palmer, Burns and Bulman, 2004) 148
Reflective Practitioner (Schon, 1984) 32, 76
reflective practitioners 32–3
  autonomous 55
reflective skills 7, 81, 82
reflectors (type of learner) **133–4**, 136f, **137**
registration (professional) 5, 21, 40, 126
  renewal 3, 58, 82, 84
  requirement to keep a profile xiii, 1, 2, 3, 38, 113
regulations 70
regulatory bodies 138
rejection 108
relationships 30, 51, 112, 147
  professional value 54
reports 71, 72, 103, 104, 121
research 72, 145
  lifelong learning 13–14
  published 81
research and development 27
research funding 139
researchers 134, 148
residential care 17
rhetoric 117

risk   112, 137
Rogers, A.   114, 119
Rogers, C.   117–18
Rogers, J.   116, 117
role play   66, 111, 134
Rouillard, L.   145
Rowland, F.   147–8
Rowntree, D.   144

Scally, M.   145
Schon, D.   32, 76, 80, 85
   two types of reflection   77
school teachers   149
science   112, 148
sculpture   29, 50, 104
Second World War   86
Sector Skills Development Agency   107
secure accommodation   17
selectivity   70
self appraisal/self-assessment   **8–9**, 12, 82,
   90, 105, 116, 144
self-awareness   7, 30, 118, 145
self-knowledge   146
self-management   145
Seven Habits of Highly Effective People (Covey,
   2001)   144–5
   Application Suggestions   145
Sheckley, B.   78
Sheckley and Keeton's learning cycle   78, 79,
   79f
short stories   71
shortages   14, 17
Shuttleworth, A.   xiv
significant events   82, 83
significant other   114
skills   xvi, 14, 18, 24, 26–7, 29, 33, 34, 41,
   43, 45, 46, 52, 55, 59–65, 65f, 71–4, 77,
   94, 95, 99t, 102, 103, 105, 106, 113,
   115, 118, 123, 127, 134, 142
   mix issues   17
   personal   40, 145
   updating   21, 25, 126
small group work   122
social activities   30
social care   xiv, 94, 127, 139
   advances   128
   continuing professional development
      21–2
   integrated   17
   performance culture   17
   PEST analysis   137, 138
   profiles and portfolios   **16–22**
   standards   **19–21**
social care assistants   xiii
Social Care Institute for Excellence   96
Social Care Register (2003–)   19
social care staff   24, 25, 26, 27
social inclusion   16, 24
social justice   21
social life   53
social services: national objectives   16
Social Services (England)   16
social situations   109
social work: international definition   20–1
social workers   xiii
Sophocles   65

standards   95
   social care practice   19
   social services   16–17
statutory bodies   xv, **2–5**
Stephenson, S.   85, 88
Strategic Health Authorities   16
strengths   82, 92
students   7, 71, 117, 119, 148
   empowerment   144
   pre- and post-registration programmes
      84
study days   14
study programmes   11
study skills/techniques   147
   annotated bibliography   **143–4**
Successful Manager series   145
SWOT (Strengths, Weaknesses, Opportunities,
   Threats) analysis   125–9, 137, 138

taking stock   **49–58**
   case study (Marian)   50–1
   focus on personal and professional
      development   52–5
   interests and aspirations   50–1
   lifelines   53
   preparation   55–8
   professional values   54–5
   real reasons for developing a profile   50,
      51, 52
   reflecting on experiences   49–52
talents   145
Taroule, J.   47
Teach Yourself with Open Learning (Rowntree,
   1993)   144
teacher education   147
teaching   117, 149
Teaching as Learning: An Action Research
   Approach (McNiff and Whitehead, 1992)
   148
team leadership   8
team-building ('key skill')   99
teams   20, 27, 33, 133, 134
   multidisciplinary   **34**, 72, 91, 138
teamwork   25, 60f
   'key skill'   36
technologies   13, 127, 139
television   25, 51
terminology   **xv, 5, 23–36**, 106–7
   'confusion'   28
   continuing professional development
      26–8
   credit frameworks   **35**
   experiential learning   **30–2**
   glossary   **36**
   key skills   **35–6**
   learning outcomes   **33–4**
   lifelong learning   **23–4**
   lifelong learning and work   **24–6**
   multidisciplinary teams: challenge for CPD
      34
   personal development planning   **34**
   profiles and portfolios   **28–30**
   progress files and personal development
      planning (HE)   **34**
   reflection   **32–3**
testimonials   59, 72, 73, 74, 104

theories   63, 64, 66, 111, 134
theorists (type of learner)   **134**, 136f, **137**
theory   112, 133, 146
thinking   136, 137, 145
thoughts   81
   private record   48
time   xv, 41, **44**, 59, 60, 81, 83, 101, 103,
      119, 121, 122, 123, 128
   reflective diary   **85–6**
time management   **55–7**, 61f, 69
   family commitments   56
   grid   57
   prioritisation   56–7
   social life   56, 58
   study   56, 57
   unforeseen events   58
   working life   56
TOPSS, see Training Organisation for the
      Personal Social Services
trade unions   99
training   10, 11, 18, 24, 25, 31, 40
   formal   21, 62
   informal   21
   social work   19
training materials (evaluation criteria)   147
Training Organisation for the Personal Social
      Services (TOPSS)   17, 22, 96, 106
training outcomes   17
travel   51
treatment (new types)   13, 26
trust   47, 90
truth   6, 137
tutors   117, 119, 122, 139

uncertainty   112, 114
understanding   99–100t
unemployment   147
UNISON   7
United Kingdom Central Council for Nursing,
      Midwifery and Health Visiting (UKCC)
      1, 7
   auditing compliance with CPD standard
      3
   portfolio requirement   2
   replaced by NMC (2002)   3
universities   8, 19, 126
US Air Force   86
Using Experience for Learning (Boud, Cohen
      and Walker, 1993)   136

values   19, 21, 64, 114
   grids   55
   personal   54
   professional   **54–5**
video tapes   29f, 29
voluntary sector   16
voluntary work/activities   51, 104, 109, 110,
      127

Walker, D.   36, 83–4, 92, 124, **146**, 149
weaknesses   59, 82
websites   96

Business and Technical Education Council
      (BTEC)   107
City and Guilds   107
credit frameworks   35
Department for Education and Skills
      13
Department of Health   28
Edexcel   107
Guernsey: Institute of Health Studies   9
key skills   99
Lifelong Learning   24
National Occupational Standards   97
Nursing and Midwifery Council (NMC)
      8, 10
National Open College Network (NOCN)
      100
National Qualifications Framework (NQF)
      101
National Vocational Qualifications (NVQs)
      98
personal development planning   34
Qualifications and Curriculum Authority
      (QCA)   106
Sector Skills Development Agency   107
Training Organisation for the Personal
      Social Services (TOPSS)   17, 106
Weil, S.   148–9
welfare reform   16
Welsh National Board: Professional Profile
      Folder (1991)   4
What Colour is your Parachute? (Bolles, 1998)
      144
Which Way Now? (Wright, 1996)   146
White, L.   143
Whitehead, N.   148
Whittaker, P.   149
withdrawal   114
work   51
   stress-free   54
work commitments   95
workbooks   42–3, 143, 148
workforce planning   17
working conditions/hours (professional values)
      54
Working Together – Learning Together: A
      Framework for Lifelong Learning in the
      NHS (2001)   19–20
   core values and skills   24
workplace   147
Wright, B.   146
writing   12, 32, 146
   fruits   82–3
   informal   46
   'permanent record'   82
   and reflecting   **82–3**
writing skills   43, 48, 58, 59, 60, 61f, 73,
      74–5, 120, 143
   formal and informal   45
writing style   40, 121
Wyatt, J.   xii

Youth Offending Team   17